INVERSION THERAPY

INVERSION THERAPY

RELIEVE LOWER BACK AND SCIATICA PAIN, IMPROVE POSTURE, AND REVOLUTIONIZE YOUR HEALTH

Includes simple plans for making your own slant board

MIA CAMPBELL

Disclaimer: The breathing routine and information in this book also appears in *The 10-Day Skin Brushing Detox* by the same author.

IMPORTANT

Don't practice inversion without consulting your physician or other health professional if you suffer OR HAVE SUFFERED from any illness, disease, or health problem. For many people it is safe and highly beneficial but there are health problems that can be made worse by inverting. Don't take a chance as you may have an undiagnosed condition. See your physician first.

There are three health conditions which mean inversion could be particularly dangerous: CARDIOVASCULAR DISEASE, GLAUCOMA, & HIGH BLOOD PRESSURE. So, if you have any of these, inversion may be out of the question for you at this time.

You should also avoid it during PREGNANCY, if you have CANCER, FRACTURES, a HERNIA, a SURGICAL IMPLANT, OSTEOPOROSIS, or INNER EAR problems.

By the same author:

The 10-Day Skin Brushing Detox

The easy, natural plan to look great,
feel amazing & eliminate cellulite

Why Henry VIII Got Fat

Secrets we can discover about
weight-loss from famous 'big' people

For Kat

CONTENTS

☙❧

INTRODUCTION

☙❧

THE SILVER FOX[1] BOUNCED INTO THE STUDIO, cheerful and confident, making the presenter look insipid and ill in comparison. He climbed onto a tall, swinging contraption and strapped himself in by the ankles. Then he relaxed, swung backwards and hung upside down for a few minutes, before doing dozens of sit-ups. He was talking the whole time, without getting out of breath.

It was incredible. Then he revealed his age – over 60. He had the figure of a man half his age and stamina to beat many athletes.

---

[1] Definition = attractive older man. His name is Roger Teeter and he founded one of the companies that makes inversion equipment, Teeter Hangups.

He credited it all to inversion therapy and explained that the machine – called an inversion table - had cured his crippling bad back. He said the inversion table could bring many people relief from back pain by relaxing tense muscles and decompressing the spine.

It made sense. The disks between the bones (vertebrae) of the spine are quite soft and gravity naturally compresses them over the years. It's one of the reasons we often lose height as we age (the other is dehydration). Decompressing your spine by lying or hanging upside down allows the disks to expand. It also reduces nerve pressure and allows the spine to realign if it has been off to the side a bit!

My [then] husband and I both suffered from sciatica and really painful backs so ordered one of the inversion tables soon after seeing it demonstrated on the shopping channel. The machine was actually **very** good. Well made, easy to use, and effective. Until then, we had been visiting osteopaths and chiropractors regularly – spending a lot of money. Inverting stopped us needing external help!

I found that I was unable to use the table as often as I needed to, sadly, because it hurt my ankles. They had been injured in a bad car wreck some years before. The bar to hold me onto the inversion table was in the exact location of the pain in my ankles and, even though it helped the pain in my back, I wasn't able to cope with the extra pressure on my ankles very often (I was able to take up inversion again a few years later, as I will explain later on!).

My husband got good use out of the table, though, and it did help his bad back a lot – until we decided to sell our table because of lack of space due to our growing family. They are quite big and we found it hard to store.

After my husband and I split up my back problems got worse. Stress has a lot to do with pain and the divorce was stressful – worrying about the effect it was having on the children, coping with reduced finances, dealing with things I'd never dealt with before (spiders!), etc. We hold a lot of stress in our bodies and that restricts blood flow, reduces mobility, and introduces pain, which causes more stress and sets up a vicious cycle.

Then along came the man who was to temporarily become my fiancé, Andrew. He has restless leg syndrome, which is often worse if he has had to stand for a while. He loves archery and has to stand for that, so his restless legs are a problem, not just an occasional niggle. A restless legs sufferer can turn into a zombie because constantly moving legs mean constantly interrupted sleep.

I told him about inversion therapy and the table I used to have. He said he would be reluctant to use an inversion table because he had had back surgery a few years previously and didn't know if full inversion – where you are actually suspended completely upside down – would be a good idea for him. He thought partial inversion might be okay.

There's a difference between full inversion and partial inversion. Full inversion means being at 90°, head down, feet straight up. Partial inversion is any angle less than that.

Research done by Alf Nachemson[2], M.D., of the University of Goteborg, Sweden, suggests that 60° inversion is as far as you need to go for your spine to be fully decompressed. Some people just enjoy going to full inversion – it is a pretty cool feeling!

People get inversion tables mixed up with gravity boots. Using gravity boots, you have to hang completely upside down; with an inversion table you start off upright and tip back until you're at the angle you want to be. Beginners often start by lying horizontal and just tipping back a little until they get used to the feeling. It's like being a kid again, hanging upside down from the wall bars in the gym!

After learning more about inversion, Andrew became convinced of the benefits of it but his physician agreed with him that using an inversion table might not be the best thing. So he decided to make a slant board.

A slant board is a board that you prop up at one end and lie on. What you prop it on determines the angle of the incline. Many people use a coffee table or armchair.

The benefits of inversion can be enjoyed from as small as a 20° incline. 20° is actually quite a shallow angle, so it's easy to prop up a board to get that degree of incline.

---

[2]   Alf Nachemson was a pioneer in the area of spine health. The National Library of Medicine hosts many of his clinical research studies.

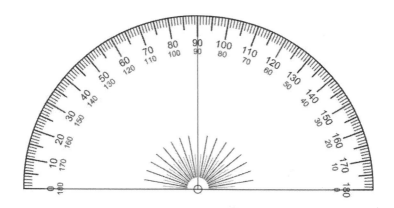

On the protractor above, 20° is the second large segment up on the left. So on a slant board your feet would be at 20° and your head would be almost at 0°, just above the floor. It hardly feels like inversion at all but it is still having a decompressing effect.

After lots of drawing, measuring, sawing, hammering, and sticking on of Band Aids, we came up with our own version of a slant board. It's a wooden one, covered with a piece of carpet. It won't win any design & style awards but it sure helps my sciatica and Andrew's restless legs. It doesn't hurt my ankles and it isn't too much for Andrew's back. It can be used with one end propped up on a couple of bricks, for a very small inversion, or on an armchair for a steeper incline.

As an aromatherapist and health coach, I am often asked for my opinion on health techniques and equipment. Once people got to know that I practice inversion myself, lots of them became interested. Having only used it myself, I wasn't about to recommend it without finding out more about who should and shouldn't invert, so I decided to thoroughly research inversion therapy. Along the way I found out that it has many more benefits than I had realized and also the health conditions that mean inversion should **never** be tried.

It's been an interesting journey and one that makes me feel even better about doing inversion myself – especially for its preventative and anti-aging effects. I'm quite evangelistic about it now as it is so easy and simple but it has such profound effects.

This book is the result of my research and I have included easy plans so that you can, if you have any ability with a saw, make your own inexpensive inversion device - a slant board. Or you could find someone who is willing to make it for you!

As with anything, it is best to get a medical professional's approval before starting something that could impact your health. A physician, physical therapist, or nurse who deals with you regularly and knows your medical history is the best person to approach. Tell them that you're thinking of trying inversion therapy. If they don't know what that is, tell them it's lying with your feet higher than your head. That'll give them a funny mental picture!

UPDATE: January 2018

My daughter and I did a two-year roadtrip in an RV around North America, between 2015 and 2017. It was a fabulous experience but it was pretty hard work, physically. We both started feeling the strain about a month in and ended up in various chiropractors' offices. My daughter had thrown her shoulder and neck out, I had recurring problems with my back and neck.

There's no substitute for a good professional's care, of course, but I didn't want to spend most of the roadtrip in doctors' offices so, after checking with the latest chiropractor that we were okay to invert, I ordered an inflatable slant board online. Within a few days of it arriving, we were both feeling much better - with more energy and vastly reduced pain. The slant board stayed inflated in our 'bunkhouse' (second bedroom) and we used it nearly every day to ward off pain and problems and help us destress after long journeys.

I now recommend inflatable slant boards to anyone who travels a lot. Ours fitted in the bottom of a suitcase easily for flying home and we use it as our regular board instead of needing a large piece of machinery or wooden slant board. It's also ideal for people who live in small apartments - or RVs!

1

WHAT IS INVERSION?

☙❧

THE DEFINITION OF 'INVERT' IS TO PUT something upside down. Inversion therapy involves putting your feet higher than your head. There are multiple reasons for wanting to do so, one being to counteract the negative effects of gravity on the body.

Physicians have been experimenting with inversion since the time of Hippocrates. The father of medicine himself used a combination of ladders and pulleys to remove weight from his patients' spines in 400BC.

It may go back further than that, though, as yogis have used inverted postures for thousands of years. The headstand and shoulderstand are examples of inverted poses and they have some similar benefits to inversion therapy. They don't, however, decompress the spine as efficiently as is done when inverting using a table or slant board. That's because when you do a headstand or shoulderstand, the spine is still being compressed by gravity - just the other way up! Using an inversion table/board means that your spine is supported while inverting and gravity can act to decompress your spine, using the weight of your head and upper body - in a similar way to how traction is used in hospitals.

Inversion is a type of traction – which means *drawing apart*. In the bad old days torturers used racks to secure their victims by the hands and feet and stretch them until their joints dislocated. Someone must have come up with the idea that this kind of stretching could be used to benefit, not hurt, people and started to use traction in hospitals. It is generally used to straighten broken bones or to relieve pressure on the spine or neck. In the old days it was common to see a line of beds in an orthopedic ward with all sorts of things attached to them to add a sustained mechanical pull to a broken bone.

When my son was three he slipped and broke his femur (the long bone in the thigh). It snapped in two, with both ends protruding past each other through his skin (it hurts to even think about it now). For it to set properly, the doctors had to pull both ends apart so they were straight again and in the right position to heal. They did that manually and then put a Thomas[3] splint on, which used gentle traction to keep the bones apart. This was great, because my son was able to come home, with the splint, rather than lie for weeks in a hospital bed with a weight attached to his foot.

So medics are very familiar with the idea of traction and modern versions of it are still used for some fractures. Inversion tables are sometimes used in hospitals, to treat problems caused by spinal disk compression. Instead of using a weight or splint to provide the traction, they invert patients and let gravity do the pulling. It is easier and less stressful for the patient.

Fast-forwarding to the 20th century, naturopath Dr Bernard Jensen was responsible for introducing inversion therapy to his patients, using a slant board.

In the 1960s Dr. Robert Martin, a California-based chiropractor, osteopath and physician, developed the 'Gravity Guidance System'. He was ahead of his time and came up with ways of upending his patients to reverse the effects of gravity, which can cause compression of the spinal disks, among other things.

In his 1982 book, *The Gravity Guiding* System, Dr Martin maintains that inversion is good for mental health too, improving concentration and memory.

---

[3] Named after Hugh Owen Thomas, the Welsh surgeon who first described it in 1875. It reduced the death rate from femur fractures from 80% to 8%. Source: The Bone & Joint Journal

He says:

> *The brain operates 14% more accurately when your body is in an inverted or inclined plane.*[4]

Inversion therapy became more mainstream in the early 1980s and started to be subject to research. Some of it was negative – which is just as important as the positive research.

Drs. Klatz and Goldman published a study in 1983 that raised concern about people with a history of hypertension, stroke, or cardiovascular disease practicing inversion therapy, as well as cautioning the elderly to be careful.

This was misreported in the media as inversion therapy being dangerous and *causing* strokes. That wasn't the truth - the physicians had been talking about specific illnesses and about full inversion.

Dr. Goldman published a second study two years later to try clarify the earlier report, and the misreporting.

He insisted that the 'risk' of stroke from inversion therapy had been exaggerated and that there had been no reports of stroke or other serious injury from practicing inversion therapy. He even said that there is

---

[4] Dr Robert M Martin, *The Gravity Guiding System*. Gravity Guidance, Inc. 1982.

more risk of cardiovascular disease in standing posture and while weightlifting.

The Evidence For Inversion Therapy

In the 1990s inversion therapy started to become accessible to more people as the cost of good quality machines reduced.

It also became the subject of more research[5], mainly into using inversion therapy for the reduction of back pain and avoidance of surgery. Things are often done for monetary reasons and this was a good one – employers spend a lot of money paying people who can't work due to bad backs!

One of the rare recent studies into the benefits of inversion therapy was published in 2012. Newcastle University in England studied patients with sciatica due to disk protrusion. They found that:

> *"Inversion therapy decreased the need for an operation in sciatica due to single level disk protrusion to 23% as compared to 78% in the non-inversion group."*[6]
>
> Pilot randomized trial,
> Newcastle University, UK

---

[5] The research since is limited. Once inversion therapy had proved itself, no-one seemed willing to put funding into proving it further!

[6] http://research.ncl.ac.uk/nctu/documents/backswing/poster.pdf

One of the researchers in that study, Professor David Mendelow, estimated that inversion therapy could save the UK £80 million (over $110 million) a year in unnecessary surgeries.

The researchers also saw a potential secondary benefit of inversion therapy being a reduction in the need for rehabilitation following surgery.

While inversion can help back pain and other ailments, its effects generally aren't permanent – you have to keep doing it. That isn't an issue for most people but it's worth pointing out that you don't just decompress your spine one or two times and hope that will do. I find that I need two or three sessions per week. My fiancé uses inversion therapy before and after every archery event that he attends, as well as whenever his legs give warning signs of impending restlessness.

My healthy, strong, 23-year-old daughter mainly uses inversion for an entirely different reason, as we'll see later when we look in more depth at some of the unexpected benefits of inversion therapy.

More and more health-care providers now allow for the use of inversion as a treatment for spinal issues. It is worth pointing out, though, that inversion should *only* be done under an expert's supervision if you have something wrong with your spine. They are in the best place to assess if it is putting too much pressure on your spine, increasing your blood pressure too much, or affecting any other medical conditions you may have (diagnosed or undiagnosed).

If you don't have anything wrong with your spine, you could use inversion as a very effective preventative measure against future disk compression and height loss.

Should We Invert When There's Nothing Wrong?

Yes, both to avoid potential problems in future and as a health-promoting habit.

Even when we are lying down, there is pressure in the disks of the spine. Fonar, the inventors of magnetic resonance scanning, have a chart on their website[7] that shows the different intradiscal pressure values when doing various activities.

There is most pressure when lifting, bending forward, and walking. There is also pressure when doing **anything else**! Lying down, laughing, twisting, sneezing, sitting, slouching, climbing stairs... everything causes spinal pressure. Interestingly, jogging exerts less pressure on the disks than walking.

One of the worst things we can do – and a lot of us do it regularly – is to sit slightly bent forward. That exerts more pressure than standing or even standing slightly bent forward. Yet how many of us sit like that most of our working days, bent towards a computer? That's quite scary for our future back health and aging.

---

[7] http://www.fonar.com/news/061206.htm

Younger people are experiencing back and neck problems and much of their pain can be traced back to their habit of using smartphones and gaming devices. Not only are they putting pressure on their disks, they are heading for neck problems and chronic headaches.

The average human head weighs between 5 and 11lbs. However, when we lean forwards, the weight of the head seems heavier to the body. That's because it isn't perfectly balanced at the top of the spine anymore[8].

Dr Adalbert I Kapandji, author of the medical textbook *Physiology of the Joints, Volume III*, says:

> *For every inch your head moves forwards, it gains 10lbs in weight, as far as the muscles in your upper back and neck are concerned, because they have to work that much harder to keep the head (chin) from dropping onto your chest.*
>
> *This also forces the suboccipital muscles (they raise the chin) to remain in constant contraction, putting pressure on the three suboccipital nerves. This nerve compression may cause headaches at the base of the skill. Pressure on the suboccipital nerves can also mimic sinus (frontal) headaches.*
>
> A I Kapandji, MD

---

[8] If your ears aren't over your shoulders, you are learning forwards – or backwards!

So our habit of leaning forward makes a lot of extra work for the muscles in our upper backs and necks – giving us 'mysterious' headaches and sinus problems. But it can get worse. Habitual tilting forward of the head can pull the spine out of alignment, cause muscle strain, pinched nerves, and herniated disks.

This is serious stuff, yet many of us habitually hunch over laptops, smartphones, and tablets. It isn't only electronic devices that cause problems, though. Even reading a book or leaning in cooing to your baby as you push his pram can do the same thing.

I bet you're sitting up a little straighter after reading that, I know I am! Those people who told you to sit up straight when you were younger? Turns out they were partly right. There is more pressure on the disks if you are deliberately trying to sit up straight, though, so it is best to sit in a relaxed but upright posture. If it helps, try thinking of lengthening your neck up towards the ceiling. It actually feels good.

There is even an increased amount of pressure on the spinal disks over the course of a night's rest – from 0.10 mpa (pounds force per square inch) up to 0.24 mpa after 7 hours. That indicates that mornings are a great time to do some inversion, soon after you get up.

Otherwise, those poor disks are permanently under pressure, there's no let-up. Over time, they get more and more compressed and less and less able to cope with doing their job as shock absorbers for the vertebrae that they hold apart. This can cause neck and back pain, sciatica, and loss of mobility and flexibility.

The spinal disks have tough outsides but soft insides and they *do* react to the constant pressure that they are put under. In a baby, the average spinal disk is made up of 80% water but the disks degenerate over time, becoming dehydrated and stiff. They are then far less able to cope with the rigors of everyday life – the bending, twisting, sitting (more pressure), and even lying down.

They can even leak and cause the surrounding nerve roots to become inflamed – which means pain, big-style.

People think spinal disks have their own blood supply but they don't (they don't have many nerve endings either). That means that they aren't able to heal themselves as well as other parts of the body which are well supplied with blood.

So it's important to keep the disks healthy and not let them get too compressed. Especially as, without their support, the vertebrae can be subject to compression fractures, leading to chronic back pain and, possibly, deformity or at least misalignment of the spine.

One of the things you can suffer is a herniated disk, where the disk bulges into a nearby nerve root. The pain is generally felt elsewhere, depending on which part of the spine is affected, or it could be felt as numbness or weakness. It can be felt in the shoulders, neck, arm, hand, etc. You can imagine that this can really affect what you are able to do with your body – it can cause complete disability.

An added problem is that pain or numbness can lead to muscle weakness. That's because we tend to move less when things hurt, so our muscles get weak through lack of movement and then become susceptible to wasting and further weakening.

This is serious stuff yet few of us do anything to ward off future problems with our spines. It's not all bad news, though, because of inversion therapy

Lying on an incline – with the head below the feet – reduces the pressure in the spinal disks, sometimes to zero. It gives the hard-working disks a rest and allows them to plump up back to their normal size and become better at their shock-absorbing task. Therefore the vertebrae are less likely to be damaged, full range of motion is kept, exercise is possible, and muscles remain strong. Instead of a vicious cycle downwards into pain, reducing the pressure in the spinal disks means a victorious cycle upwards!

Several important studies have demonstrated this, including the Nachemson[9] study that I mentioned earlier. That was one of the first studies to prove that there is residual pressure inside the disks even when lying down and that traction equal to 60% of body weight while lying down almost eliminated the

---

[9] http://fonar.net/pdf/spine_vol_24.No.8.pdf

pressure. According to Canadian Chiropractor[10], that kind of traction is attainable by inverting to 60°.

There are other benefits of inversion therapy, apart from its decompressing action on the spinal disks...

---

[10] http://www.canadianchiropractor.ca/content/view/1461/38/

2

THE BENEFITS OF INVERSION THERAPY

CRSR

AS I HABITUALLY DO, WHEN I SAW THE inversion guy on TV, I got the wrong message. He said that he used to be in such pain with his back that every morning he had to crawl out of bed to the bathroom and stay in the shower for 10 minutes, until the heat of the water unclenched his muscles. Now he practices inversion, he no longer needs to do that.

That was the message I was supposed to get, that inversion is good for bad backs. Instead, I thought, "Long steamy showers, they sound good!" They did do some good, I found that a long, hot morning shower helped my back pain tremendously. My husband, though, was of the opinion that buying an inversion machine would save money on the electricity and water bills. He was probably right!

A hot shower or bath does help some painful conditions (not all) but it can also be very debilitating. Baths are terrible for me in the mornings, I'm like a sloth all day if I start off with a bath instead of a shower.

The Canadian website *Save Yourself*[11] has some interesting things to say about hot baths:

> ***They don't call it 'heat exhaustion' for nothing: enduring intense heat can be tiring.***

A hot shower or bath, while providing some relaxation to the muscles, can be counter-productive because it excites the nervous system. You may notice your heart pounding after a very hot shower or bath.

Inversion relaxes at the same time as energizing. Just a couple of minutes on my slant board gives me an energy boost while decompressing my spine and reducing – usually eliminating – the pain from my lower back and sciatic joint by decompressing my spine.

---

[11] http://saveyourself.ca

Around half of the people who practice inversion regularly do it to relieve some sort of back or neck pain. It is particularly helpful for sciatica, which often doesn't respond well to other methods of treatment.

This raises difficulties, though, because while inversion can help alleviate the pain of some health problems you really you shouldn't try inverting if you have a health condition without consulting your physician.

However, many medical professionals are very open to the idea of inversion therapy, having seen it used successfully in hospitals and back pain clinics. Your physician may suggest something other than inversion, perhaps traction. A study on inversion concluded that:

> *"Although mechanical traction has been used for centuries, only gravity assisted traction (inversion) offers an effective means of achieving pelvic traction at home."*[12]
>
> Gianakopoulos, G, et al: Inversion Devices: Their Role in Producing Lumbar Distraction

So hospitals and clinics may have different ways of getting a similar result.

Do ask for your physician's opinion before trying inversion therapy yourself. It may be that he/she needs

---

[12] Gianakopoulos, G, et al: Inversion Devices: Their Role in Producing Lumbar Distraction. Arch Phys Med Rehabil 66: 100-102, Feb 85.

to check that you don't have any sign of an underlying, undiagnosed condition that would make inversion contraindicated.

Easing Back Pain

Back pain can be caused by many different things but, if a cause has been ruled out by a medical professional, it is often due to posture or habits. Compression of the disks is one of those habits. Bad backs used to be caused by heavy work – farmers, builders, laborers. Then, they were caused by heavy lifting.

Often, it was due to lifting while leaning forward. In that position there is a *lot* of uneven pressure on the spinal disks. If you add to that the weight of the object being lifted and – possibly – a slight twist as you straighten up, your back is in trouble. That's why health & safety posters warn us to lift with our legs, not our backs. That means we should bend our knees and not lean forward when picking the object up. Too many of us disregard these notices as being bossy and irrelevant – until we slip a disk or find ourselves immobile due to muscle spasms in the back.

Nowadays it is common for people to injure their backs without doing anything at all. People will say they have no idea how it happened, they weren't lifting anything or twisting. Look at how we tend to work, though. We sit at computers, *leaning forwards all day*. Our disks are under more pressure than the farmers of old who were out digging fields all day – at least they got to straighten up occasionally.

I suffered from excruciating headaches and neck pain for a few weeks. My doctor couldn't find a cause and just prescribed stronger and stronger painkillers. One day my son came into my office and frowned. He said, "Do you know you should have your laptop screen at eye level?" Yeah, I did. I had been an IT teacher - I should have been practicing what I preached!

I was using a laptop frequently, for many hours a day. Unless you prop a laptop up on something, it is far lower than eye level, so you have to look *down* at it all the time. I was putting the disks in my neck under constant pressure. That pinched the nerves and the surrounding muscles went into spasm so I had a combination of neck and head pain that had been sending me crazy.

My son ordered me a laptop stand that same day and it arrived the next day. The day after that my headaches and neck pain stopped. If I had continued using my laptop in the way I had been, I doubt that the pain would have gone away so easily. I could have done long-lasting damage.

Inverting will help the pain if you have damage like that because it relieves the pressure on the disks. We do have to look at the cause of our pain rather than just trying to relieve it, though. Our disks are under constant pressure simply due to gravity. If we add to that pressure by leaning forwards habitually, we are going to be in trouble one day.

When I'm working to complete a book I work long hours, sometimes 16 hour days. My family keep an eye on me because they know I have a tendency to slouch forwards when I'm concentrating intensely. They nag about my posture and I used to get irritated ... until I did the research for this book! I was horrified at how much pressure we put our backs under simply by our posture and habits.

If you have back pain, inversion could bring you wonderful relief. Unless you tackle the cause of the pain, though, it will just keep coming back.

Improve Posture

The spine naturally has a gentle 'S' shape but we tend to alter that through poor posture habits. When inverting, gravity pulls the spine back into its 'S' shape.

This can, eventually, correct poor posture habits as you start to realize how much better you feel when you stop slouching, leaning, and sitting oddly.

Easing Sciatica

Sciatica can also have numerous causes, e.g. a pinched nerve, a herniated or slipped disk, narrowing of the spinal canal, piriformis syndrome (a spasming muscle putting pressure on the sciatic nerve). Sufferers usually don't care what has caused their pain (which is often felt in the leg rather than or as well as the lower back), they just want to get rid of it. It can be very painful. When you have sciatica it feels like you don't get any rest, ever, as you can never get comfortable.

What is generally happening is pressure or compression of a nerve – the sciatic nerve. The sciatic nerve is long – the longest nerve in the body. It goes through the pelvis, glutes, and legs. That gives it a lot of places where it could get trapped!

The main cause of sciatica is a slipped disk. One of those disks that we have been talking about as being decompressed during inversion. If you can decompress your disks you have a very good chance of easing or eliminating your sciatica.

Medical treatments for sciatica vary from rest and anti-inflammatory drugs through a range of interventions such as injections in the spine and surgery. Physical therapy is sometimes offered and can be very effective. It aims to reduce pressure on the sciatic nerve via stretching, exercise, and massage to ease tight muscles.

One of the studies[13] done on inversion therapy involved people who were unable to work due to back pain (from various causes, including sciatica). They focused on 175 patients and, after just eight inversion treatments, 155 of them were able to return to work.

---

[13] Sheffield F.: Adaptation of Tilt Table for Lumbar Traction. Arch Phys Med Rehabil 45: 469-472, 1964.

The study reported:

> **"Significant improvements in a variety of diagnosis including spondylolisthesis, herniated disks, lumbar osteoarthritis with sciatica, and coccygodynia."**
>
> Sheffield F: Adaptation of Tilt Table for Lumbar Traction

Sciatica can go away on its own but if it lasts longer than a few days, it does need to be checked by a physician. If he/she gives you the okay, it could be well worth you trying inversion as a non-invasive, inexpensive, easy way of relieving or eliminating your pain. Watch your posture as well!

Avoiding Surgery

Severe back pain suffers often end up needing surgery. One of the things surgeons can do for back pain is to fuse problem disks together. That can take away the pain but adds problems by reducing mobility – you can find yourself unable to twist.

Numerous studies – including the Newcastle University study[14] mentioned earlier – have demonstrated that inversion therapy, used as part of a treatment program,

---

[14] http://research.ncl.ac.uk/nctu/documents/backswing/poster.pdf

can reduce the need for surgery. It is popular in many clinics because it is so effective and inexpensive.

It may be that you could avoid surgery by using physician-approved inversion therapy. You may even be able to find a clinic that offers inversion therapy as part of an overall treatment regimen.

Reducing Muscle & Joint Pain

Backs aren't the only parts of the body that get painful as we age, work, or slouch. Muscles also feel the effects of gravity, as well as wear and tear. They can also go into spasm, which is very painful.

Muscles can also become tense due to misalignment of the spine. Inversion is very effective at stretching and invigorating muscles, which helps the spine to realign and lengthen. That increases circulation and helps to reduce overall tension in the body, thereby helping the joints as well.

When the spinal disks are decompressed it increases blood and oxygen flow all over the body due to the release of compression on the veins and arteries that run around the disks.

Preventing Loss Of Height

Gravity isn't always a bad thing, ask any astronaut - that Canadian guy[15] seems pretty accessible! NASA reports that prolonged zero gravity affects the body in many ways. Zero gravity won't affect many of us though so we don't need to be concerned about the effects of inversion temporarily reducing the effects of gravity.

Instead, over the course of a lifetime, gravity has some very negative effects on us. The biggest problem – as we saw in the last chapter - is that it compresses the disks that sit between the vertebrae of our spines, causing us to shrink.

Elderly people are often dismayed to find that they have lost height – sometimes up to as much as three inches. Men seem to find this particularly upsetting.

The National Library of Medicine reports that:

People typically lose about 0.4 inches every 10 years after age 40.

Height loss is even more rapid after age 70.

Medline Plus, National Library of Medicine[16]

---

[15] Chris Hadfield, the astronaut who spent five months on the International Space Station. He's on Twitter: @Cmdr_Hadfield

[16] http://www.nlm.nih.gov/medlineplus/ency/article/003998.htm

Loss of height is something that regular inversion can prevent or reduce. NASA tells us that astronauts usually come back to earth at least two inches taller than before they left. So we can assume that regularly inverting could – even if temporarily – help us to grow a little taller.

It seems that we are so affected by gravity because we have such a lot of water in our bodies. Some sources say around 78% at birth, dropping to 55-60% in adults and even less in the elderly. Compare a baby's wonderfully pudgy hand to an elderly person's, which will often be thin, dry, and lacking in elasticity.

Keeping ourselves hydrated - especially as we get older - is very important. It is made worse by the fact that we often override our thirst instinct throughout our lives because we don't want to have to be running to the bathroom, and the fact that the thirst mechanism is often much reduced in elderly people.

Elderly people are also more likely to exist on packaged, pre-prepared foods, especially if they have health problems. Standing, cutting up vegetables, and lifting heavy pans are all difficult when you are in pain. Packaged foods have generally been processed, stripping them of vital nutrients and *water*.

If you are considering taking up inversion therapy, you might want to consider working on your hydration at the same time. The double-whammy could have a big effect on your health and level of comfort.

Anti-Aging

Pain, lack of mobility, and loss of flexibility are things we associated with old age (although they can happen earlier). Many of them are caused by the natural effects of gravity over the years compressing the spinal disks.

The spinal disks also suffer from becoming more and more dehydrated as we age, which is interesting because a lot of things that we associate with age are also associated with dehydration, such as:

➤ Dry, sticky mouth

➤ Sleepiness

➤ Dry skin

➤ Headache

➤ Dizziness/lightheadedness

➤ Confusion

➤ Constipation

➤ Lack of sweating

➤ Sunken eyes

➤ Shriveled skin that lacks elasticity

There are a lot of myths about drinking water. No-one has ever claimed to have come up with a scientific reason for the '8 glasses of water a day' rule. If you eat a lot of high water-content foods (fruits and vegetables), as well as drinking smoothies, juices, and other beverages, adding a further 8 glasses a day could take you into the 'too much water' camp.

Too much water is as bad as too little and can even result in hyponatremia, where the body's electrolyte balance is dangerously disturbed (even fatally, in rare cases, such as marathon runners).

So how should you go about making sure that you don't get dehydrated? It is surprisingly easy and it has nothing to do with thirst, which can be a bit unreliable. We tend to over-ride our thirst mechanism – either by ignoring it completely or by eating instead of drinking. It also reduces with age.

Instead, let's take advice from the world-renowned Mayo Clinic[17], which says that it is safest to go by your urine output:

> *Thirst isn't always a reliable gauge of the body's need for water, especially in children and older adults. A better indicator is the color of your urine. Dark yellow or amber color usually signals dehydration.*

Improving your hydration can also be helped by eating more vegetables. Accompany that with reinvigorating your whole body through inversion and it could have an amazing effect on your health.

---

[17] http://www.mayoclinic.org/diseases-conditions/dehydration/basics/symptoms/con-20030056

The other anti-aging benefits of inversion include protection against dementia, reduced depression, and increased blood flow to the brain.

Does this mean that we've hit on the fountain of youth? I don't know for sure but, as it is non-invasive, inexpensive, easy, and fun to do, I'm placing my bet on inversion giving me a big anti-aging boost. I certainly feel a lot better since I started inverting regularly.

Reducing Stress

As I mentioned earlier, stress causes a vicious cycle of pain, stress, and more pain. One of the reasons for this is muscle spasm, often in the neck and shoulders or the back. It can result in horrible pain in the area affected, as well as other areas, resulting in headaches, insomnia, and [understandable] mood changes.

We ignore the dangers of stress to our cost. It really is a killer. A friend of mine went through a horrendous situation that meant she had to leave her home and move to another country with two young children and no income. Over the following years her health declined to worrying levels. When she had a medical examination to try to find the cause of crippling headaches, the surgeon asked her when she had suffered a serious blow to the head. She replied that she never had. He insisted that she must have been in some sort of severe accident but she hadn't. Eventually he asked if she had suffered extreme stress, which of course she had. He nodded, saying that the stress could have caused the same injuries to her brain that he thought a serious blow to her head had caused. Stress can have serious *physical* effects on the body.

Inversion is relaxing and it reduces stress by giving a feeling of wellbeing, increased blood circulation, and improved removal of toxins by the lymphatic system[18]. It eases physical stress on the joints, disks, muscles, and nerves and increases oxygen throughout the body.

General Wellbeing & Prevention

David Coulter is huge fan of the inverted postures that are practiced in yoga. He knows a lot about the human body, having received a Ph.D. from the University of Tennessee and taught anatomy at the University of Minnesota for 18 years.

He explains that inverting allows fluids from tissues in the lower extremities to drain. You might think that lying down what have the same effect, but it doesn't.

He says:

> *"If you can remain in an inverted posture for just 3 to 5 minutes, the blood will not only drain quickly to the heart, but tissue fluids will flow more efficiently into the veins and lymph channels of the lower extremities and of the abdominal and*

---

[18] For more on how to help the lymphatic system, see my book *The 10-Day Skin Brushing Detox* http://amzn.com/B00HYQ5L98

> *pelvic organs, facilitating a healthier exchange of nutrients and wastes between cells and capillaries."*
> David Coulter, Ph.D.

This is great news for the body. It means it has to work less hard. It's quite hard work pumping blood down to the feet and back up again. Giving it a helping hand through inversion makes sense.

Decompressing the spine, oxygenating the tissues, stretching and releasing joints and muscles, and reducing the pulse rate all have very beneficial effects on the *entire* body.

The gentle stretching and releasing of the joints and muscles can even ease frozen joints. Once they are released, exercise can again be done to increase mobility and circulation and reduce pain and the likelihood of further injury.

A few years ago, I managed to tear a ligament in my shoulder, just by reaching behind me in the car to open the back window for the dogs. It was a horrible pain. A few visits to a local sports therapist sorted it out with some massage and sound wave therapy.

However, it happened again, sending me into the arms of a physiotherapist near my home (I couldn't drive to the sports therapist!). The pain was truly horrendous, I couldn't get any rest and had to resort to high-strength analgesics from the hospital – something I hate doing.

The physiotherapist did some gentle movements and sound wave therapy and gave me exercises to do at home. I asked if I would now have a permanent problem with that shoulder and why it was so weak.

He explained that most people don't do the exercises they are given. They are given them for a reason, because if the sore area isn't kept mobile the blood supply isn't as good, muscles can get weak, and you can end up with a frozen shoulder (or whatever joint is affected). That's serious because it is much more difficult to correct.

He went on to explain that some parts of the body are less richly equipped with blood vessels than others and that exercise helps to get fresh blood to those areas.

The physiotherapist was right, I hadn't kept up with the exercises that I had been given last year. You can be sure that I have now! They're actually really simple, just moving and circling my arm to keep things moving in there and using inversion to decompress everything and encourage fresh blood flow to areas that are less well-fed with blood. It's part of my 'preventative' strategy so that my muscles, disks, and joints stay limber and healthy to prevent future injuries.

Tendons and ligaments have very little blood supply, which is why they can take a long time to heal if they are injured – longer than fractures sometimes. They simply aren't getting the nutrient supply that they need to repair (such as protein).

I'm quite excited about the fact that simply inverting is helping to get blood to parts of my body that don't have lots of blood vessels. Knowing that I am improving the way that nutrients and oxygen are sent to those areas and increasing the removal of wastes from them makes me feel really good about inverting.

If you have a history of being easily injured, inversion could be a big help by improving both the rate at which you heal and the likelihood of you being injured in future.

The website *Be Well Buzz* reports that the US Army Physical Fitness School found that:

> *Soldiers who inverted regularly with inversion equipment suffered fewer joint related injuries or back muscle pain and healed more quickly from joint compression damage.*[19]

So inversion is very good at preventing injuries, as well as helping heal them.

Help Insomnia

Inversion's relaxing effects definitely help insomniacs. This is largely due to the decrease in muscle tension, as the muscles are naturally stretched by the effects of

---

[19]   http://www.prweb.com/releases/2012/3/prweb9345588.htm

gravity pulling the other way than they are used to going!

If you suffer from insomnia, you could make inverting a part of your before-bed routine. It will act as a signal to your body that it is time for sleep, as well as relaxing you.

Faster Healing

Inverting regularly means that you are increasing the oxygenation of the cells and organs. It can speed up the overall healing processes and detoxification.

Improved Digestion & Elimination

Many people who invert regularly report better functioning of their digestive organs and increased energy. That's because regular inversion, due to decompressing the internal organs, can lead to improved functioning of the internal organs, especially the kidneys, liver, and pancreas.

Internal organs can move around or prolapse (particularly the large intestine). Inverting allows them to move back into place.

If you suffer from abdominal fat – known as visceral fat – you probably also have fat around your internal organs. Losing the weight is important and, once you are down to a weight to begin inverting, you will be able to help your internal organs rearrange themselves back to where they were before the fat started squishing them and nudging them aside.

Even something like Irritable Bowel Syndrome (IBS) can be helped by inversion. Partly, this is because of the relaxing effects of inversion but it is also because of the gentle yet effective decompression of the internal organs.

IBS often accompanies back pain, so it is interesting that inversion helps both. They may be more connected than we think.

Weight Loss

This is a subject close to many people's hearts – me included! I've had a battle with my weight since my car wreck stopped my athletic hobbies. Being unable to do the exercise I had been used to made me pile on weight and my inability to walk meant that I wasn't able to shift it.

Inversion can help weight loss by improving the health generally, giving you more energy, and reducing pain – thus enabling you to exercise more.

One of the mental blocks that prevents many people from losing weight is the dread of having sagging, loose skin afterwards. Be assured that this only happens for people who lose massive amounts of weight very quickly – for example after gastric band surgery. It seems to worse for women after menopause, as the skin is less elastic.

Often, the health dangers of remaining obese far outweigh the risks involved with losing weight quickly. One of the problems is indeed the possibility of being left with sagging skin. That's because, when a body is very overweight, the skin has been stretched beyond its capacity to bounce back quickly.

Bariatric surgery[20] is often the last chance an extremely overweight person has of surviving. The rest of us have more time to lose the weight slowly enough to give the skin chance to catch up with what's going on!

With the mental block of being left with sagging skin removed, you may have more success in your weight loss journey. Here a few things you can do to ensure you remain healthy while losing weight:

➤ Skin brushing. Just get a skin brush and start, it has an amazing effect on the whole body. It tones up the skin and underlying muscles, so helping the skin bounce back as you lose the weight. Skin brushing also stimulates collagen production and gives the skin a healthier appearance.

➤ Eating/drinking 7-10 cups of vegetables a day. This is advice from one of my health heroes, Dr. Eric Berg[21]. He says it will not only supply the body with much-needed potassium, it will stop cravings and help regulate the appetite.

---

[20] Bariatric = surgery performed on the stomach and/or intestines to help a person with extreme obesity (BMI of 40+) lose weight. Source: MedicineNet.com

[21] http://www.drberg.com/

➢ Keeping to a well-balanced diet. That means lots of fruits, vegetables, slow release carbohydrates (e.g. sweet potato, brown rice, quinoa), plant proteins (e.g. lentils and beans), and good sources of fats (e..g olive oil, coconut oil). These will supply the macro and micro nutrients your body needs and will: help your skin recover and regain its elasticity; keep your intestines working well due to the fiber content; give you the energy you need to keep going.

➢ Rehydrating yourself. The best way is the Mayo Clinic way – by monitoring your urine output. Some days you may not need to drink very much water, especially if you have been eating a lot of fruits and vegetables, juices, smoothies, etc. Other days, when you resort to processed foods because you're on the go or in meetings, you may notice that you need a lot more water.

➢ Taking up moderate exercise and health habits. Inversion therapy, gentle exercise such as swimming, rebounding, yoga & Pilates can give you back your mojo and help get your metabolism back to normal. Some light weight training can really help – by toning your muscles and increasing your metabolism. Metabolism is the rate at which your body functions. The more efficiently it processes things, the better. That means it will process your weight-loss more effectively, your skin elasticity, your muscle repair. Weight training is the golden key to lasting weight loss, as the improved muscle tone and function increases the body's needs for calories – so you get to eat more **and** keep the weight off!

> Reducing your stress levels. If you are an adrenal body type, you will be prone to weight gain due to raised levels of the stress hormone, cortisol. Reducing stress itself is very difficult but it is much easier to control your *response* to stress. Practicing relaxation, doing meditation, or just going for a gentle walk can all help control the stress response.

I'm not a weight-loss expert but Dr. Berg is. Check him out - do the [free] body type quiz on his website and watch his numerous [free] informative videos on YouTube[22]. He has some books[23] available, too, which are excellent.

If you're worried about me raving about him, be assured that I don't know him personally and I'm not gaining anything by recommending him. I just respect his immense knowledge and desire to help others.

Improved Hormones

We can tend to see hormones as the banes of our lives. When we have teenage acne, we blame our hormones; when we get unnecessarily angry we say we have too much testosterone; when we go through the rollercoaster of menopause we blame our diminishing estrogen.

Yet hormones (aka the endocrine system) are simply chemical messengers that act on different aspects of

---

[22] http://www.youtube.com/user/Bergdiets?feature=watch
[23] http://www.amazon.com/Eric-Berg/e/B001K8HRVG

bodily processes. While it is true that unbalanced hormones affect us in [very] negative ways, balanced hormones make us feel absolutely wonderful. One of the ways we can help our bodies to keep hormones in balance is through inversion.

Inverting stimulates the pituitary gland, the main endocrine gland which helps balance the entire endocrine system. The pituitary is responsible for secreting and storing hormones and stimulating other glands that control hormones. Improve the pituitary and you improve the whole endocrine system.

Better Menstruation/Menopause

[MEN, DON'T READ THIS YOU MAY FIND IT YUCKY!]

The jury is still out on whether or not women should invert while actually menstruating. Partly, this is because of outdated ideas that blood loss is helped by gravity and that inverting could send the blood the wrong way. That's now been disproven but many experienced yoga teachers still caution against inverting during blood flow.

Anecdotal reports from women who have inverted while menstruating (either by doing yoga or using an inversion machine) reveal some negative effects. It seems it can interrupt menstrual flow, only for the period to resume some days later.

Some women fear developing endometriosis, where bits of womb-like tissue appear outside the womb and bleed during menstruation (it's painful, I've had it). This has also been debunked as there isn't an opening at the top of the womb for the tissue to go through, although flow can go back up the fallopian tubes. This is known as *retrograde menstruation* but studies[24] have shown that it can occur naturally in up to 90% of women, many of whom never go on to suffer from endometriosis.

However, the study's conclusion does say that that **quantity** of retrograde menstruation seems to have a bearing on whether or not a woman develops endometriosis (as well as several other factors).

Another explanation for the idea of not inverting during menstruation comes from the idea that the womb becomes quite heavy during the period. That's because by the time it is ready to start bleeding the lining has become thick (ready to nourish a growing baby). It is thought that inverting could cause the ligaments that hold the womb in place to overstretch.

In the end it comes down to personal choice and comfort. It's more important to listen to your own body that to the opinions of others. You may find it comfortable to avoid inversion during the first couple of days of blood loss, though, when the flow is at its heaviest.

On an interesting note, I sailed through menopause with hardly any symptoms. I think it was partly due to

---

[24] http://humupd.oxfordjournals.org/content/8/1/84.full.pdf

regular inversion helping my hormones and stress levels but I can't prove it.

[OKAY GUYS YOU CAN CHECK BACK IN NOW]

Improved Intelligence

This is a controversial benefit but many people report sharper thinking and even improved memory after taking up regular inversion. There may be something in it, as the increased blood and oxygen flow to the cells in the brain will benefit it.

The author of *How to Increase Your Intelligence*, Win Wenger, believes that 'upside down activities' help intelligence by this very thing – increasing the oxygen supply to the brain.

The reverse is certainly true. People with illnesses that slow down the oxygen supply to the brain (such as hardened arteries) do experience a reduction in cognitive function.

Better Mood

Inversion can even improve the mood. One reason will no doubt be its effect on stress and hormones, but it could also be due to increased blood flow to the brain.

Better Complexion & Hair

COMPLEXION

In a 1984 edition of the comic of *Archie's Girls Betty & Veronica*, Betty is seen hanging upside down on an inversion table[25]. As the girls are usually fighting for their hero Archie's affections, I think we can safely assume that writer intends us to guess they have discovered the beauty benefits of inversion.

The beauty industry is worth billions of dollars. Women alone spend $426 billion a year on beauty products, with 17% of them using three to four products a day.[26] Many of these creams and lotions are for covering up or reducing the effects of aging and skin damage. That's something that inversion does without any cost at all! The beauty industry doesn't want us to know that inversion can make us look great, though, as they don't earn anything from that.

Inverting brings increased blood flow to the upper part of the body – the parts that can need the help of anti-aging creams, especially the face, neck, and décolletage. The blood brings nutrients and oxygen, which plump up and refresh the skin, improving the exchange of wastes. Inversion also boosts the lymphatic system, which helps clean up and get rid of cellular debris.

The result is firmer, healthier skin that has a youthful glow. If this is what you are after, keep an eye on your

---

[25] http://en.wikipedia.org/wiki/Gravity_boots
[26] http://shine.yahoo.com/shine-beauty/insane-amount-money-women-spend-beauty-192900715.html

hydration too as that will give an even better combined effect.

HAIR

Years ago, I read an article by a woman who attended a yoga class. She remarked to the tutor that she found it strange that his hair style changed so much. He would have a long ponytail one week, cropped hair the next and, within a short space of time, his hair would be long again. He told her it grew quickly because he did inverted postures (such as the headstand and shoulderstand).

It makes sense, as being upside down would bring increased blood flow to the head, more nutrients, oxygen, and improve the transfer of wastes. I didn't think it would be quite as effective as it is, though, until my daughter started doing inversion.

She always had beautiful long hair until she suffered from anorexia for a number of years. Part of the body's response to lack of food is to shut down what it considers to be non-essential systems. One of the first things to go is hair health. My daughter's formerly glorious hair became dry and lackluster. It broke easily, faded, and refused to grow. Her body was far too busy keeping her alive at that time to worry about something as insignificant as her hair. To her, though, it was hugely important, as it is to many people - as anyone who suffers from hair loss could confirm.

Now, please bear in mind that our experience is purely anecdotal. We didn't conduct a controlled experiment and it did coincide with my daughter getting better, and using oil blends that I made up. However we are convinced that inversion had a big effect on the *speed* of her hair growth. It probably wouldn't have worked as well if she hadn't started giving her body the nutrients it needed but it did seem to grow much more quickly than we expected. She can now sit on it. It has gone back to its rich, natural color, and has an enviable gloss. Now that she is eating more nutrients, she is getting them to her head more efficiently by inverting!

An article on a leading hair blog confirmed our deduction. The Longing4Length blog has an article[27] titled, 'Inversion Method for Hair Growth – One Inch in One Week'. The writer said she had tried a type of inversion in her youth:

> *"Instead of just brushing my hair with one hundred strokes, I would do so while leaning upside down off the side of my bed ... now of course I wasn't taking length pictures then and I can't remember how long I kept up the ritual but it seems to me that I remember noticing a difference in my hair's thickness and length."*
>
> Longing4Length Blog

---

[27] http://longing4length.com/2013/07/inversion-method-for-hair-growth-one-inch-in-one-week.html

In the article, she reposted a photo of someone else who had tried inversion and the difference in the length of her hair is clear. The comments on the post from other people who have tried inversion for hair growth are also interesting.

If you are going for hair growth, here are a few tips from my daughter:

➢ The 100 brushes a night thing is counter-productive if you have curly hair. It will cause frizziness and pull out a lot of hair. Brushing once a day is enough to detangle or style – preferably with a natural plant bristle brush. Use a comb at other times, one with widely-spaced prongs.

➢ Brushing is also intended to stimulate blood flow. You can get the benefits of that by massaging **gently** with your fingertips and by inverting. Stick to inverting if your hair is very fragile. Massage and brushing can damage it and cause more hair loss.

➢ Only use products on your hair that you wouldn't mind eating! I'm joking of course, but try to get products that are made of natural ingredients. They are less harsh and less drying on your hair and scalp.

➢ Rinse your hair with cool water after washing. It is an old-fashioned tip but one that works by improving blood flow and resealing the cuticles. It reduces frizziness and stops your hair getting greasy too quickly.

➢ Consider adding a little cider or white vinegar to your rinse water. It helps balance the hair's pH.

➢ Sleep on a silk or satin pillow case and wash it frequently (e.g. once a week) in mild detergent.

➢ Do inversion for a couple of minutes once or twice a day.

➢ Use coconut oil as a leave-in mask once a week. Add other goodies to the oil if you have them to hand – avocado is very nourishing, so is egg yolk. Black castor oil is a great addition if you want to stimulate growth. Apply shampoo directly to your hair before rinsing it off. If you use water first it makes it harder to remove.

➢ Ensure you are getting good nutrition. Make sure that everything that passes your lips will give you nutrients, not make you lose nutrients. In general, if it came from a factory, it won't have many nutrients left in it. If you struggle to eat, home-made vegetable juices are a great way of getting a boost of nutrients without lots of calories or heaviness.

➢ Don't use elastic bands on your hair. Use only wrapped bands and hair accessories that have soft edges. Try to leave it loose frequently.

➢ Try to avoid heat styling your hair – or at least give it a couple of days off a week from heat! The easiest thing is to braid it and leave it to dry naturally.

Varicose Veins & Hemorrhoids

Some illnesses are definitely made worse by gravity, generally those that are caused/aggravated by standing, such as varicose veins and hemorrhoids.

Store workers, nurses, and other people who have to stand for long periods are likely to suffer from varicose veins, as are pregnant women and those suffering from obesity. People with constipation, pregnant women, and older people are more likely to suffer from hemorrhoids.

VARICOSE VEINS

You can often see varicose veins on the backs of people legs in summer. They are painful, enlarged and twisted veins near the surface of the skin. They are caused by weaknesses in the veins and in the valves that are inside them. The valves are there to prevent backflow of blood but they can get congested. So blood flow is slowed and backed up and pressure builds.

Inversion helps by relieving the downwards pressure and helping the valves in the veins to empty.

Again, it needs approval from a physician before starting because some vein problems are caused by fragility.

HEMORRHOIDS

Hemorrhoids are similar to varicose veins in that they are swollen or inflamed veins in the anal canal. They can be inside or protruding outside the anus. The exact cause of them is not known but they are known to be more common in people with constipation, dehydration, a low fiber diet, pregnancy, and 'straining' on the toilet.

Inversion helps via its anti-gravity and relaxation effects and by decompressing the internal organs. The decompression of the disks of the spine also benefits the entire body.

Recovery After Workouts

Those who do high impact exercise know the feeling of total exhaustion that can hit afterwards. It can happen to a lesser extent to those of us who are less fit and active, just from light activity. It all takes a toll on the body and can be worse if our spines are slightly misaligned. Inversion helps by decompressing, stretching, and relaxing the muscles, joints, disks, and vertebrae, allowing them to rehydrate and replenish themselves.

Inversion also stimulates the lymphatic system to get rid of wastes more quickly and efficiently. It can reduce the next-day pain after an intense workout and help you keep at peak performance if you have an active professional or hobby.

Some inversion experts call this the *lymphatic wash*, which is a lovely expression. The Energy Center[28] describes why this works very well:

---

[28] http://www.energycenter.com/grav_f/benefits.html#train

> *"Intense muscle activities cause muscles to become sore. This is due to the buildup of large amounts of lactic acid and cellular debris in the muscles. Unlike the cardiovascular system, the lymphatic system has no pump.*
>
> *Only the alternate contraction and relaxation of muscles move lymphatic fluid 'uphill' through capillaries and one-way valves to the upper chest for cleansing. Inverting the body so that gravity works with, not against, these one-way valves helps to push the lactic fluid up to the chest. The faster the lymphatic system is cleared, the faster the ache and pain of stiff muscles disappears."*
>
> www.energycenter.com

Are you convinced of the benefits of inversion therapy? There are even more, reported by lots of people, and the benefits you get will likely be very individual to you. At the very least, though, you will get the tremendous boost of reversing the life-long effects of gravity on your body.

Natural medicine pioneer Dr Bernard Jensen once said:

> *"There is not a single disease in which gravity does not play a part."*

> Dr Bernard Jensen

An interesting – if controversial – statement but one that is quite encouraging if you are able to do inversion therapy.

Don't rush straight in, though, because there are some people who shouldn't invert...

3

WHO SHOULDN'T INVERT?

CRITICAL: ⌘

HEALTH, FITNESS, AND DIET BOOKS ALWAYS include disclaimers that readers should check with their physician before embarking on any regimen that could affect their health.

That's never been more true than with inversion. Not that it is dangerous, it is because it affects so many body systems. For example, it can temporarily increase blood pressure, so you would want to check if that would be safe for you. You don't necessarily have to suffer from high blood pressure now for that to be relevant.

Seriously, DO check with your physician before starting inversion therapy. That's the case whether you have any existing/diagnosed illnesses or not. They will often do a quick check while you're there.

That said, there are some illnesses that mean you really can't do inversion therapy.

> *"Your heartbeat slows and your blood pressure increases when you remain inverted for more than a couple of minutes — and the pressure within your eyeballs jumps dramatically. For these reasons, you should not try inversion therapy if you have high blood pressure, heart disease or glaucoma."*
>
> Edward R. Laskowski, M.D. [29]

Heart, Stroke, & Circulatory Issues

Any illness involving the heart or circulation means that inversion is not recommended. That includes people who are taking anti-coagulants, people who have had a stroke or TIA, and anyone who suspects they may have had a TIA but hasn't been diagnosed. Symptoms include paralysis, difficulty speaking, and memory loss.

---

[29] http://www.mayoclinic.com/health/inversion-erapy/AN01614

Hypertension/High Blood Pressure

This is because inversion affects the heart rate and blood pressure. If you already have high blood pressure, inverting could put it up to dangerous levels.

Eye Problems

If you have any eye problems you should check with a physician or eye specialist before trying inversion therapy. Glaucoma in particular is a problem because it means there is already higher pressure in the eyes.

Pink eye, conjunctivitis and retinal detachment – or any other inflammation of the eye - are also contraindicated for inversion.

Bone Problems

Inversion is a type of traction, a sort of mild version of being on a medieval rack! For that reason, if you have weak bones, then you could be hurt by inverting. So osteoporosis, spine injury, recent fractures, skeletal implants, and other bone issues all mean that inversion could aggravate the condition.

Hernia

A hernia happens when an internal part of the body protrudes through another part, usually a muscle. Often this is caused by pressure in the abdomen. As inversion therapy puts upward pressure on the body, it could make a hernia worse. If you have a history of hernia, it is best to check with your physician to see if inversion would be helpful or harmful.

Disorientation Problems

Until you know the cause, and your physician has given you the go-ahead to try inversion, it is best to avoid it. Disorientation – including balance problems, middle ear infections, dizziness, and feelings of fogginess – can have many causes. Finding out the cause is important and waiting until any infection has passed is vital.

Obesity

This is hard because people who are obese are often in pain and desperate to find something to improve their health. Inversion seems like a good idea because it reverses all the impact the joints get. However, if you are obese there are some very good reasons why inversion therapy could be dangerous for you. Being obese is a risk factor for numerous illnesses, including circulatory problems. Often these go undetected for a long time. So you could have a slightly raised blood pressure or heart problem and inversion could put extra pressure on your body that it just doesn't want to cope with.

Added to this is the problem that many inversion systems have a weight limit, so you may struggle to find one to accommodate you.

You can get some of the benefits of inversion by simply raising your feet and legs, though. You can find big wedge-shaped cushions in many stores. Pop one of these under your lower legs (wide-edge at your feet, narrow edge towards your knees).

Pregnancy

Pregnancy puts a lot of pressure on the body. It may be that you would benefit from a gentle incline on a slant board to take some of the pressure off your abdominal and perineal muscles, but it is vital to get a physician's approval first.

Certainly don't invert if you have any pregnancy complications, without checking with a physician first.

According to the Cure Back Pain and Sports Injury Clinic websites, inversion therapy should not be used by pregnant women. The Energy Center warns that pregnant women should get a physician's approval before inverting. Inversion therapy could have a negative effect on the mother or baby depending on the mother's condition and the baby's stage of development.

Prescription Drugs

If you are on any drugs that thin your blood (e.g. Warfarin or aspirin), you shouldn't invert. The very fact that you are on them indicates that you are at risk of something – possibly stroke – which means inversion wouldn't be good for you.

Spinal Injury/Surgery

If you are or have been under the care of a spinal specialist, neurosurgeon, or orthopedic surgeon, you need to be very careful with your spine. It may be possible for you to invert but only with the very clear say so of your physician and probably under their watchful eye. If you don't or can't get their approval, it *really* isn't worth the risk.

⊂ʒ४⊃

If you do suffer from any of the conditions above and inversion is ruled out for you by your physician, there is something you can gain from the research into the benefits of inversion.

It is that **sitting or standing while bending forward is one of the worst things you can do in terms of the pressure on your spinal disks**. Just stopping yourself doing that will help your health.

4

DIFFERENT TYPES OF INVERSION

CRICO

MACHINES, BOOTS, YOGA, BOARDS – THEY can all be used to do inversion. Which is best for you? Your budget, the size of your home, and your inclinations will help you decide.

The main options are:

- ➢ Yoga – inverted postures
- ➢ Gravity boots
- ➢ Inversion table
- ➢ Inversion chair
- ➢ Slant board

There are some other pieces of equipment that can be used to get some of the traction benefits that inversion gives. Let's have a look through the different options and possible costs involved.

Yoga

Yoga is described by Yoga Australia as:

> *"An ancient system of philosophies, principles & practices derived from the Vedic tradition of India & the Himalayas, more than 2,500 years ago. Yoga cultivates health and wellbeing (physical, emotional, mental, & social) through the regular practice of a range of many different techniques, including posture and movement, breath awareness and breathing exercises, relaxation and concentration, self-inquiry and meditation."*
>
> Yoga Australia

The word 'yoga' comes from two words, one meaning 'to yoke' and the other 'to concentrate'. It is sometimes translated as 'union with the divine'. Others prefer to think of it as a type of moving meditation.

THE POSES

Each type of yoga uses different poses and names for poses but most of them do inverted postures that many of us might associate more with childhood activities!

The most popularly-known are the headstand – where your body is upside down, resting on the crown of your head; the shoulderstand – where you are upside down but your head, neck, and shoulders are on the floor, with your hands bent at the elbows, propping your upper back up; and the plow (or variations of it), which is similar to the shoulderstand but with the legs swung further over the head, not straight up.

Yoga is an increasingly popular hobby, with over 20 million people practicing regularly in the United States alone. Not everyone is a fan though.

RELIGIOUS OBJECTORS

Due to its association with Hinduism, some people would rather not do it. Atheists sometimes have a problem with yoga classes. Having gone along to participate in a form of exercise, they are often shocked at the spiritual elements of yoga. People of other religions also struggle with the fact that some of the poses in yoga have them bowing to Hindu deities.

One person who won't do yoga is Laurette Willis[30], who grew up in a yoga-loving home. She was spiritually hungry and was open to, and tried, everything:

---

[30] http://www.todayschristianwoman.com/articles/2005/march/truth-about-yoga.html

chanting, crystals, tarot cards, psychics, Habbalah, Taoism, etc. She spent time in an ashram, a Hindu yoga retreat and taught yoga herself.

Eventually she found what she was looking for (although, as a committed New Ager, would have been horrified if anyone had suggested it!) and became a Christian. That caused her to give up everything that she had been doing before which had caused her unhappiness – which included yoga. To her, it was very much linked to the New Age practices which had not brought her the peace that she had been seeking and it went against her new beliefs.

She now heads up the PraiseMoves[31] exercise regime, which is dedicated to teaching a Christian alternative to yoga. She explained why to BBC News[32]:

> *"The sound 'om', chanted in many yoga classes, is meant to bring students into a trance so they can join with the universal mind. And the 'salute to the sun' posture, used at the beginning of most classes, pays homage to the Hindu sun god."*
>
> Laurette Willis

She no longer wanted to pay homage to a Hindu deity, but to her own God.

---

[31] www.praisemoves.com
[32] http://www.bbc.co.uk/news/magazine-25006926

Other religions agree. Yoga is only allowed in [Muslim] Iran (where it is very popular) if it is referred to as a 'sport' and classes concentrate on the physical benefits, without including meditation, projection, or other more spiritual practices. In Malaysia, a 2008 religious ruling banned yoga in five states.

Some yoga practitioners insist that it is not associated with Hinduism (or no longer associated with it, if it once was), while others are horrified at what they see as the Westernization and dumbing-down - spiritually - of yoga. While the debate about whether yoga is intimately linked to Hinduism rages on, people of other faiths with bad backs may want to consider alternative ways of getting the benefits of inversion, even if they do other yoga postures.

SAFETY OBJECTIONS

William J. Broad is a senior writer at *The New York Times* who has won every major science journalism award (in both print and television). He also won the Pulitzer Prize twice and is the author or co-author of seven serious-titled books.

Not the sort of person you imagine getting his 'Om' on but he's been practicing yoga since 1970. He wrote a book that rattled the cages of a few yogis called *The Science of Yoga: The Risks and the Rewards*.

He is used to delving into scientific papers and when he began to research yoga he did so with *"a sense of wariness"*. The book that was the result of his research is fascinating, unearthing not only numerous health benefits but also 'waves of injuries'. He says:

> *"Overall, the risks and benefits turned out to be far greater than anything I ever imagined. Yoga can kill and maim – or save your life and make you feel like a god. That's quite a range."*
> William J. Broad

Sadly for yoga fans, the exercises that he uncovers as having the most potential for injury are the inverted postures. Broad says his research has caused him to change his own yoga routine (he remains a fan). He says he has *"de-emphasized or dropped certain poses"*.

Some yoga experts have realized the dangers and either adapted poses or warned of the risks. One is physician Timothy McCall, who is the medical editor of *Yoga Journal*. He wrote on the *DailyCupOfYoga* website:

> *"Some poses, like headstand, shoulderstand, and lotus, are inherently risky if not done with good anatomical alignment. Some people have contraindications to doing certain poses. So, for example, someone who has poorly-controlled high blood pressure or diabetic retinopathy should avoid headstand and other inversions as they could precipitate a retinal hemorrhage."*
> Timothy McCall, M.D.

In light of both Broad's and McCall's considerable experience and credibility, it looks like the inverted yoga poses can be somewhat risky. Even the YogiTimes website[33] agrees:

> *Being upside down has its risks, however. Just as there are safety concerns that prompt many communities to ban jungle gyms and monkey bars from their playgrounds, there are reasons why chiropractors, physiotherapists, and massage therapists – among others – would prefer that we not balance on our heads and necks.*
>
> YogiTimes

To be fair, many of the problems associated with inverted yoga postures are particularly risky – like inversion therapy generally – only to those with existing health conditions. The same things that preclude inversion therapy - such as glaucoma, high blood pressure, and cardiovascular disease - rule out inverted yoga postures. Although there is the added problem in yoga of some of the postures actually compressing the disks in the neck (e.g. the headstand).

There are things we can learn from yoga, though, whether or not we decide not to try it ourselves.

---

[33] http://www.yogitimes.com/article/yoga-inversion-inverted-asanas-poses-benefits-risks-safety-spine

Timothy McCall admits to having suffered from a bout of thoracic outlet syndrome (TOS).

TOS is a relatively rare condition that can cause pain in the neck, shoulder and arm, as well as numbness or tingling in the fingers – often accompanied by a lack of ability to grip properly – and a restriction in circulation to the extremities, sometimes causing discoloration.

The Mayo Clinic describe TOS as occurring when:

> *"The blood vessels or nerves in the space between your collarbone and your first rib (thoracic outlet) become compressed.*
>
> *This can cause pain in your shoulders and neck and numbness in your fingers."*
>
> Mayo Clinic[34]

TOC can be caused by car accidents, repetitive activity, poor posture, obesity, or pregnancy but occasionally - as was the case with Timothy McCall – it can be caused by yoga practice.

McCall admits that it was his practice of the headstand (also known as the plow pose) and shoulderstand that played a role in his suffering from TOS.

He says that:

---

[34] http://www.mayoclinic.org/diseases-conditions/thoracic-outlet-syndrome/basics/definition/con-20040509

> *"Part of it could also be blamed on my own stubbornness … just before I developed intermittent numbness and tingling in my right arm, I'd been increasing my headstands up to 10 minutes a day, even though that was more than I could comfortably do. I was allowing an external goal suggested by someone else – not my own body's feedback – to dictate when I came down. I now believe that at the moment (or just before) you lose that balance of effort and ease in the pose, if your breath is rough, or if it just doesn't feel good, you need to come out."*
>
> Timothy McCall

This is important for us to remember in our inversion therapy – however we choose to practice it. Listening to your body is vital. Don't let someone else dictate the amount of time you should invert, or the angle. If it doesn't feel good, you need to stop.

If you decide on inverted yoga postures as your form of inversion therapy, the main thing to ensure is that you chose a great, experienced instructor. An experienced instructor will be able to guide you into the correct position and ensure that you stay safe.

William J. Broad advises his readers to find a highly qualified and experience yoga instructor. He explains that the Yoga Alliance's definition of a yoga teacher is anyone who has participated in at least 200 hours of 'real training' (whatever that means). That's equivalent to four to five weeks. He asks: "Would you study with a violin teacher who had trained for a month? A sculptor? A basketball player?"

He points out that Iyengar yoga requires people to have practiced the style for at least three years before applying to train as an instructor. Its teacher training is a minimum of two years and Iyengar "have redesigned some of yoga's most dangerous poses. Teacher training puts much emphasis on how to lessen the risks."

Maybe you have a fantastic, experienced yoga teacher who is knowledgeable of the potential risks and keeps your mind fully on the poses you are doing. If so, great! If not, do be careful.

ADVANTAGES OF INVERTED YOGA POSTURES:

➢ Inexpensive – can be done at home via a DVD or online course or at a class

➢ Relaxing and [possibly] social

➢ Has other benefits

DISADVANTAGES OF INVERTED YOGA POSTURES:

➢ Possible problems for those who have issues with the spiritual aspects and/or roots of yoga

➢ Some inversion poses are potentially dangerous

Gravity Boots

In the 1980 film *American Gigolo*, Richard Gere straps on a pair of odd-looking books, then leaps up and grabs a bar bolted to the ceiling. He hoists his legs up and hooks the boots over the bar, where they seem to hold on fairly precariously. He then does a series of exercises while hanging upside down. The world was introduced to inversion – and Richard Gere's amazing abs!

The only systems available to invert in the 1980s were based on Robert Martin's *Gravity Guidance System*, using gravity boots. Gravity boots became very popular and gained a reputation for alleviating back pain and headaches.

The boots themselves generally have sturdy hooks on them, which attach to a bar that's wedged onto a door frame. That may sound a bit precarious but they're robust and don't move! Some supporting bars are permanent, others can be moved.

The idea is that you strap on your gravity boots, jump or reach up and grab the bar, then swing your legs up to hook the boots over the bar.

As you can imagine, that takes a bit of effort and strength. I certainly don't have the strength to do that. If you have ever tried and failed to hang by your hands from the wall bars in a gym or children's play area, you won't like gravity boot systems.

They are much more suited to athletes, soldiers, and other physically fit people who want to get even fitter (you can exercise while hanging upside down), help recovery, and undo some of the damage they have inflicted on their bodies from all that tough exercise!

Gravity boot systems start from around $150. Amazon sell the Teeter Hang Ups EZ Up Inversion System[35] for $153. It hangs on any standard wooden doorframe. The boots – sold separately from around $99[36] – are 'one size fits most', so obviously need to be tried on before buying if you have a large or small shoe size.

I haven't tried a gravity boot system because of my ankle pain and lack of upper body strength but I have to confess that being a wimp has also put me off!

However, several people have told me that gravity boots are more comfortable on the ankles than inversion tables. Some people even use gravity boots **with** an inversion table.

One problem with gravity boots is a slight sense of panic you can feel. On an inversion table, most people can touch the floor quite easily when they rotate backwards. It gives a feeling of stability and you can rock back up to a more comfortable angle if you start to get a pounding head. You may not be able to touch the floor when hanging from gravity boots on a tall doorframe.

---

[35] Teeter Hang Ups Inversion System http://amzn.com/B000M83J5I
[36] Inversion Boots http://amzn.com/B000DLB8RU

Reporter Harry Wallop tested out a gravity boot system for the UK's Telegraph newspaper[37]. He wrote:

> *"My fingers can't touch the floor, leaving me feeling as vulnerable as a punchbag and the blood rushing to my head is unpleasantly intense."*
> Harry Wallop

So gravity boots aren't for everyone. As Wallop said, it's quite intense. Some people really like them, though. They tend to be preferred by people who are already quite fit, healthy, and athletically-inclined.

While researching this book I kept reading that the US Army use gravity boots but I was unable to track down an original source for that information. I eventually found an article tucked away in the archives of the United States Army website from October 2011. It has a photo[38] of a physical therapist lowering an injured solider onto an inversion table. So they definitely use inversion tables but I was not able to find any official reference to gravity boots.

The Teeter Hangups inversion company says on its website that their gravity boots are in regular use at the US Army Physical Fitness School in Ft. Benning, GA[39].

---

[37] http://bit.ly/danbrowninversion
[38] http://www.army.mil/article/67309/Physical_therapy_taking_ away_Soldiers__pain/
[39] http://blog.teeter-inversion.com/why-the-us-army-trusts-teeter/

It makes sense that the Army would use gravity boots for their healthy soldiers and inversion tables for the injured guys. Gravity boots are definitely more suited to people who are physically fit.

ADVANTAGES OF GRAVITY BOOTS:

➢ Takes up minimal space

➢ Good for people who want to exercise while inverting – no leg bars in the way

DISADVANTAGES OF GRAVITY BOOTS:

➢ Best for athletes and other physically strong people

➢ Not ideal if you don't already have good core strength

➢ Not for people with mobility problems

Inversion Tables

After the surge in popularity of inversion in the 1980s, one of Gravity Guidance System's sales consultants went on to develop an inversion machine that didn't require boots and a strong doorframe. That evolved into the modern inversion table.

This was a massive breakthrough as it meant that people who weren't physically strong were able to enjoy the benefits of inversion.

Most inversion tables operate by clamping down the feet and ankles. You lie on a 'table' which pivots on a fulcrum attached to a support frame (the legs of the table). This allows you to climb on comfortably in a standing position, clamp yourself on, and lean back slowly. The slowness is very important because if you suddenly swing over to full inversion it feels very weird and isn't a good idea – too stressful for both body and mind!

Instead, you can lie horizontally for a while before gradually tipping yourself backwards – aided either by the handles at the top of the machine's legs or by raising your arms over your head. The handles give an added sense of security because you know you can pull yourself back up by them if you need to. You probably won't need to, though, because you can use your arms. When lying at an angle, if you raise your arms over your head, towards the floor, and then swing them back up towards your legs, you cause the table to start to swing back up.

The thing I like best about inversion tables is the ability to change the angle of the incline so easily. Some even have a strap to prevent the board going further than you want to, when you're beginning. You feel quite safe (the frame doesn't tend to rock) and fully in control.

If you do have painful ankles, you can try adding extra padding to the ankle clamp. Old memory foam mattresses cut up are great for this! If you have any comfortable boots you could try wearing those and some people wear gravity boots.

Weight and height limits vary but generally machines aren't able to cope with people over 300 pounds in weight or over 6' 6" in height. Costs vary from around $60 to over $4,000 for commercial machines.

ADVANTAGES OF INVERSION TABLES:

➢ Feels secure and comfortable
➢ Can go to different degrees of inversion easily and smoothly
➢ Can go to full inversion (90°) easily – and slowly, without a head rush
➢ Can exercise while at full inversion

DISADVANTAGES OF INVERSION TABLES:

➢ Takes up quite a lot of room as you need space for the table to swing
➢ Not for people with sore/weak ankles or knees
➢ May be difficult to store

Inversion Chairs

These are new to me, I've never used one but I came across them when doing the research for this book. They look like a piece of gym equipment called the leg curl. They aren't widely available, it seems that they haven't become as popular as inversion tables yet, which is a shame because they have some important advantages over tables.

You sit on the chair, generally with your knees cushioned on a foam bar, and wedge your ankles between two further foam bars. Many chairs also have a seatbelt – which people love because it takes pressure off the ankles. Then you lean back and relax. Some people can find it difficult to get into the chair, because of the leg and ankle bars being in the way, so this could be an issue if you have mobility problems.

There are a couple of disadvantages. They tend to be a bit more expensive than an equivalent quality inversion table and they take up more room than a [folded] table. That said, some models are foldable.

You can't go to full inversion in a chair but, as you get full decompression benefits at 60°, that doesn't really matter. It just means you can't do much exercise while inverted – you can exercise your arms though.

If you are less than about 5' 4", you may be best to try a chair out first, rather than ordering it over the Internet as some models seem to have been made with tall people in mind!

The advantages are great, though. A chair is better for people with sore or weak ankles and/or knees, as you're not hanging from your ankles or putting pressure on your knees. There are some back conditions which make it painful to lie with the legs straight, in that case a chair is idea.

People report that they can use a chair on their own, without help, which is quite liberating. They are said to be very comfortable and feel secure and sturdy. Much less scary for beginners to inversion than a table.

They can be harder to find than inversion tables but Amazon stock them and Walmart have been known to have them in from time to time. They start from around $200.

I can't speak personally but people have recommended Health Mark as being a good manufacturer. Health Mark is a Georgia-based company. Some of their products, at least, are American made, which is a bonus!

ADVANTAGES OF INVERSION CHAIRS:

➢ Secure and comfortable

➢ Easy to use without help

➢ Less scary than a table when tipping backwards

➢ Smaller and less bulky than an inversion table

➢ Better for people with weak ankles than an inversion table but the ankles are still strapped in so not ideal for everyone

DISADVANTAGES OF INVERSION CHAIRS:

➢ Slightly awkward to get into

➢ May be difficult to store

➢ Doesn't go to full inversion

Slant Boards

A slant board is simply a long board that either has legs or is propped up on something. You can use a couple of bricks, a low stool, a coffee table, a chair, etc. It can be covered with material to make it more comfortable and give more grip, such as rubber or carpet. It is sometimes referred to as an incline board. (We're talking about a board long enough to lie on - not the desk-top boards that are sometimes used to help dyslexics write or the small incline boards that are used to stand on to help ankle stability.)

If you are at the budget end of the market for your inversion therapy, this could be for you, especially as you could even make your own slant board. A slant board is the best choice for people with weak ankles or knees or lack of space in their home.

However, if you have a problem getting down onto the floor, then you would probably find it hard to get on and off a slant board.

The biggest plus of my slant board for me is that there is absolutely no pressure on my ankles. I also have a hard time lying flat on my back without bending my knees. Lying with my legs straight for long gives me horrible back pain. On my slant board I am able to bend my knees (often one leg at a time) and still get the benefits of inversion.

One of the advantages of a slant board is that, because of the angle, most people can stay inverted for longer than they would on an inversion table (once they have got used to inversion). I've been doing inversion for years so I'm quite comfortable staying on my slant board for 15-20 minutes while doing reading a book or listening to music.

In fact, inverting on a slant board is a wonderful relaxation technique, even without considering all the other benefits that inversion brings. If you combine your sessions with some deep breathing, you will find it gives you a good feeling all over – sort of cleaned out and with more of a spring in your step.

It can be difficult to get onto a board if you have mobility issues. I do it by propping my board up at one end on an armchair, then sitting down in the middle of the board. Then I can swing my legs up and lie down.

As I said earlier, you start getting the benefits of inversion at a 20° angle so, as long as you have something you can put your board on to give you that angle, you're golden.

You can progress to a steeper angle later on, if you wish, once you're used to inverting. I use my sofa or armchair to give me about a 40° angle and that's great.

Going much steeper could start to become dangerous as there is a chance you could slip off backwards. For that reason, we have covered our slant board with carpet, which gives a great grip.

You could go further and attach some straps to the sides to use as handles, just to give you extra reassurance.

The cost of buying a slant board starts from around $50 but you could make you own for less than that.

Please don't be tempted to take the advice of some articles I have read that advise people to lie on a 'sturdy ironing board'. I haven't come across an ironing board sturdy enough to safely take the weight of anyone heavier than a 5-year old! It would be an uncomfortable and unpleasant experience. A bought or home-made slant board is much better, as well as being safer and more comfortable.

There are some wonderful variations on slant board available now, including an inflatable slant board made by Airslant[40]. It has a built-in pump so is very easy to inflate and deflate. This is the board my daughter and I used on our roadtrip and it proved worth its weight in gold! It enabled us to continue the trip, when pain could have ended it. We left our board up most of the time on the trip but now we're back we inflate it when we want to use it and it only takes a few minutes.

---

[40] http://amzn.com/B00EA1OUWE

Another type I like – but haven't used – is one made from big foam wedges. A bit hard to store, I would imagine but wonderfully luxurious!

ADVANTAGES OF SLANT BOARDS:

➢ Inexpensive – free if you have suitable materials to hand. From around $50 for commercial boards, $100 for inflatable boards

➢ Can be easier to store than large inversion machines. Mine slips behind furniture - some people have room underneath furniture for theirs

➢ Light and easy to use

➢ Less of an incline, so better for people with weak ankles or knees, or other health problems (providing a physician has agreed to inversion)

DISADVANTAGES OF SLANT BOARDS:

➢ Not suitable for people who want full inversion or to invert at a steep angle

➢ If your board doesn't have legs you need something sturdy to prop it on

➢ Not suitable for people who can't get down onto the floor

Other Inversion-Type Methods

LIKE EVERYTHING ELSE, A PHYSICIAN SHOULD BE CONSULTED BEFORE USING ANY OF THESE METHODS, ESPECIALLY YOU HAVE AN EXISTING HEALTH CONDITION OR SUSPECT THAT SOMETHING IS WRONG.

If we think of inversion as a method of traction – of taking pressure off the spinal disks – and of reversing the effects of gravity, there are several smaller, inexpensive pieces of equipment that can give some similar effects.

You won't get the full benefits of inversion therapy from these but they are excellent for helping back pain, stiffness, and problems caused by poor posture.

Anything you can do to reverse the compression in your spine is going to make you feel better.

FLEXIBAK[41]

The Flexibak is a small wooden cradle that was invented by an osteopath to ease back pain. It almost looks like part of a skeleton, made of wood. It's a compact unit, easy to store and transport – which is a huge plus for people who travel a lot. An inversion device isn't the easiest of things to travel with!

The Flexibak has 8 wooden segments of decreasing sizes, which are separated by rotating nylon rods. The

---

[41] www.flexibak.net

whole thing will twist in your hands, rather like the spine does.

The idea is to lie on the floor with your knees bent, lift your hips and then slide the Flexibak underneath you with the largest segment under your pelvis and the smallest segment pointing towards your head. What it does it tilt your pelvis up slightly – or invert it – while cradling and supporting it, taking pressure off the spinal joints, disks, muscles, tendons, and possibly compressed nerves.

There are some exercises that you can and should do while lying on a Flexibak. One of them is rocking your knees from side to side slowly. It is a very pleasant, freeing feeling, and the Flexibak's inbuilt rotation ability is perfect for assisting this. The wooden segments massage the back muscles that they support as you rock.

The Flexibak is perfect for helping lower back pain and reversing some of the effects of poor posture.

Jason Rosser, the inventor, says:

> *"Traction, movement, and pressure are the three most effective ways of easing lower back pain."*
> Jason Rosser, Osteopath
> & inventor of the Flexibak

The Flexibak does all three things: it provides traction by gently holding the vertebrae apart (without causing pain); it provides movement by the rocking motion performed while supported by the cradle; and it provides pressure on the muscles either side of the spine from the wooden segments on the cradle.

The Flexibak website also points out that decompressing the joints in the back not only helps the back itself but is good for general wellbeing and vitality.

Unlike inversion, a Flexibak can be used safely by pregnant women. It is also recommended for cases of arthritis, sports injuries, sciatica, and other lower back problems.

The Flexibak is available from **www.flexibak.net**, as well as from International distributors, for around $125.

They haven't gone through FDA approval (yet) so it isn't available from US websites or stores. It has been tested and approved by many other countries, though.

ADVANTAGES OF FLEXIBAK:

- Small and light, easy to store and transport
- Easy to use without help
- Not at all scary
- Comfortable
- Money-back guarantee if it doesn't help relieve your pain

DISADVANTAGES FLEXIBAK:

> ➢ May not be suitable for people who have had back surgery

> ➢ May be uncomfortable for people without very much body fat, or who are frail

Stability/Swiss Ball

The stability ball was first used as a medical device by British physiotherapist Mary Quinton. Mary had worked through the Blitz of the second World War. In 1942 she traveled to Malta, to help the victims of a polio epidemic there and set up the island's first physiotherapy unit. All that changed after she attended a course about a new approach to treating cerebral palsy in children.

She wanted to move into this new neuro-developmental work and initially decided to move to an underdeveloped country to help children there. However, one of the people she met on the course was a Swiss doctor, Dr. Elsbeth Kong. Dr. Kong's opinion was that Switzerland was a valuable place to offer the treatment as, not having been involved in wars, it had not developed skills in the rehabilitation of injuries.

In 1957 Quinton moved to Kong's home country temporarily and ended up staying there for the rest of her life. She worked with babies and children (and their families) who had developmental problems caused by cerebral palsy.

After it was invented by a plastics manufacturer in 1963, one of the things Quinton used in her treatment of babies was the stability ball. It was later termed 'Swiss ball' by American physical therapists who visited to find out how to use it with their patients.

You will still find stability balls in physical therapy clinics and rehabilitation units. They are also very popular in gyms now, as an exercise device.

Today's balls go by lots of different names, including: balance ball, Swedish ball, Pilates ball, yoga ball, etc. I just mean one of the really big exercise balls that you can sit on.

The ball is unstable because, as balls do, they roll. When you sit on it your muscles have to work at keeping you upright, or in whatever you position you are in. That's why Mary Quinton had such success with them with children, it helped their neuro-development by making their muscles work to keep them balanced (which made new brain connections).

A stability ball's role in helping pain comes from this instability, because your core muscles (which surround and support the abdominals and spine) have to work to keep your balance.

So it is very good at preventing back and other pain. Exercising – or even just sitting – on a stability ball is a quick way to improve core strength and reduce the risk of back injuries by keeping the supporting muscles strong.

It has another use as well. If you sit on a ball and 'walk' forward with your feet while leaning backwards, you can lie back on your ball with your head supported. Your back will be bend backwards and supported by the ball.

This won't be decompressing the spine in the way that an inversion device does, but it stretches it in the opposite way to the way you probably sit/walk the rest of the time, so it provides relief. It's a wonderful stretch that feels great and can be enhanced by stretching your arms back over your head (if you can).

Balls start from around $10.

ADVANTAGES OF A SWISS BALL:

- Light and inexpensive, easy to deflate and store
- Easy to use without help
- Comfortable and pleasant to use
- People who get headaches or who don't like inversion devices sometimes like the stability ball

DISADVANTAGES OF A SWISS BALL:

- May not be suitable for people who have had back surgery
- May not be suitable for people with a poor sense of balance

So there are lots of devices and ways to try inversion therapy. Whichever you choose, you'll need to know how to get started ...

5

GETTING STARTED

ᘒᘒᘒ

I HAVE LOST COUNT OF THE NUMBER OF independent testimonials I read while doing the research for this book. They were all from people who had been in pain and were really helped by inversion. They had nothing to gain from writing their stories, they just wanted to help other people who were struggling.

Many had been able to wean themselves off analgesics and other medications, or at least reduce the dosage.

Some were delighted at the unexpected side-benefits they experienced from regular inversion – glowing skin, glossy hair, less wrinkles, more energy.

There were also cautionary tales as well, from people who had rushed into it without checking first with their physician. I think I've gone on enough about that for now! It just isn't worth the risk.

I pored over all mentions of inversion therapy, inversion, and inverting online, in an effort to find problems that people had had with inversion. I wanted to be able to forewarn my readers, to enable you to be on the lookout for potential problems.

Lots of people do mention the only trouble that I experienced when I started inverting ... the head rush.

We simply aren't used – as adults! – to hanging upside down. It causes a rush of blood to the head and can give you a headache or sinus pain if you invert too long.

It can take up to a month to get used to inverting and not experience the head rush or headache. The best approach is to:

Start Slowly

When you realize all the benefits that inversion therapy brings, it can be tempting to jump in straightaway and hang upside down for an hour or two. Please don't! You'll get a whopping great headache and probably won't be able to stand upright for a while afterwards!

It's a bit like when you spin round in circles and it disturbs your balance. Inverting does the same. Take it slowly and you will gain the benefits rather than experience side-effects.

A minute or two is long enough for your first couple of inversions. Build up slowly to longer periods. Don't invert for longer than 5 minutes for your first month of inverting.

Start With A Shallow Incline

Use a shallow incline[42] for your first couple of sessions. Go for 20° initially. Once you are used to that, try a *slightly* steeper incline and stick with that for a few days before going further.

Aim for a 60° incline if you can, eventually, but don't force it. You will be getting many of the benefits of inversion even at 20°. You won't be achieving full decompression of your spine at 20° but, after a lifetime of being permanently burdened, your disks will be glad of any slight lessening of pressure!

When traveling, you could carry an inflatable slant board. They cost around $99 online. They only take a few minutes to inflate and deflate and fit under a bed or in a suitcase easily when not in use. They only give a small incline – around 25° - but it is enough for most people.

---

[42] Obviously this isn't possible with a gravity boots system but, hopefully, you'll have tried inverting a few times using another method before doing full inversion on a gravity boots system.

Frequency

Invert no more than once a day for the first couple of days. You can then move up to twice a day if you wish.

Most people invert daily but there are lots who invert just a couple of times a week and still enjoy full benefits.

Once you are used to inverting, you should be able to do it twice daily but I wouldn't do it more than that.

When we had our inversion table it was a bit of a hassle to drag it out from a storeroom. So we got into a routine of getting it out and inverting before bed, leaving it set up. Then we would invert next morning and put it away. We did that a couple of times a week.

With the slant board it is easier as we store it behind the sofa so it is easy to slide in and out.

It isn't for me to tell you how to run your home but do remember that lots of people buy exercise equipment that they use once and then use as a clothes storage device! For that reason I recommend to most people that they try to find somewhere that loans equipment, or where they can try it out first. If you aren't sure whether or not you will take to inversion therapy, a slant board is the cheapest method of trying it out. You could progress to a table or chair later on if you love it and it helps you.

After Inverting

Stay still for a few minutes after coming back up to let your brain and body realize what's going on. In the case of a slant board, sit up slowly or slide off onto the floor and lie there for a couple of minutes before sitting up.

One of the things that inversion does is to rehydrate parts of your body that are usually squished and slightly dehydrated. You can help that along by drinking a glass of water after inverting. Don't drink it before inverting – or close to the time you're going to invert – as it can make you feel a bit sick.

6

EXERCISES TO DO
WHILE INVERTING

ভ৪৪৩

I F YOU WATCH SOME YOUTUBE VIDEOS ABOUT inverting you could be forgiven for thinking that it's an endurance, Olympic-type sport! That's because the super-fit guys do all sorts of maneuvers whilst at full inversion. People can do amazing exercises while inverting that they can't otherwise manage. BUT you have to be very strong and healthy to do them and I would advise you to get a specialist DVD or instruction if you want to try them.

Actually you don't have to do anything other than lie and enjoy the stretch. If you want to, though, you can do a few exercises to maximize the benefits of your inversion time.

These are the simple movements that you can do on an inversion table or slant board. I'm not experienced in using gravity boots so I can't give instructions for the incredible exercise that be done using them. It seems to involve a lot of 'sit-ups' (actually lie-ups!) and twists.

Here are a few gentle movements that are both effective and easy to do on either an inversion table or slant board. Like any exercise, you don't want to attempt them when your muscles are cold, or you could hurt yourself. If you do your inverting first thing in the morning, walk around for a few minutes first so your muscles are awake. It's a good time to go and get a glass of water (perhaps with a slice or squeeze of lemon) that you can enjoy after your session:

1. Lie back to a good inversion angle (i.e. 20° or more) and relax for a minute or two.

2. Become aware of your breath and think about expanding your abdomen to allow more air in. Let your next in-breath be deep and slow, filling your lungs so that your ribs move out to the sides a little. Take a few more deep breaths before starting the movements.

3. Slowly raise your arms straight up, then back and over your head to rest them behind you – on the ground if you are on a slant board, dangling in mid-air if you are on another inversion device. Relax there for a few seconds before raising them upwards again and

lowering them back to your sides. This move stretches the abs, which is wonderful because they very rarely get stretched in this way and it is effective at toning them. Do it a couple of times.

4. Stretch your arms out to the sides and relax them there if you can for a few seconds before bringing them back to your sides.

5. Raise your arms straight up in the air, fingers pointing towards the ceiling. Raise your left arm up, as if trying to touch the ceiling, then let it gently fall back. Repeat on the right side. This is the 'shoulder reset', a Pilates move. It's good at getting our usually slouching shoulders back into the position they should be in.

6. With your arms by your sides or folded comfortably across your chest, lean towards your left side. This gives a good stretch to your right side and also elongates your back, giving some space for the disks to expand. Repeat on your right side.

7. Bend your knees so your feet are flat on the board. Let both knees lean towards the left, as far as they will comfortable (and safely!) go. Feel the stretch in your right side and hip. Bring them back to center then lean then towards the right. Bring them back to center and rest for a few seconds before repeating.

8. Bend your knees towards your chest then relax them slightly away (still bent). Your legs will be compressing and then releasing your abdomen,

which is great for stimulating activity in there! Good for constipation.

9. Put both feet on the board with your knees still bent, then raise your left leg and straighten it up towards the ceiling. Point your toe and stretch your leg more towards your chest (you probably won't be able to get close to your chest but you know what I mean!). In this position, flex and point your toes twice. Feel the stretch in your hamstrings while flexing, try to hold it for a second or two. Bend your leg again before relaxing your foot back to the board and repeating with your right leg.

10. Relax on the board for a minute or two before getting up.

These gentle exercises can be performed at any time of day. If you are performing them before bed – which is a great time because inverting before bed can help you sleep – be sure to do them slowly so you don't wake yourself up too much.

7

HOW TO MAKE YOUR OWN SLANT BOARD

ೞೞ

IF YOU WANT TO TRY INVERSION THERAPY AND don't have room in either your bank balance or your home for a commercial machine, then you might want to try making your own slant board.

You don't have to be a carpenter but you do need to know your way around a saw. If you don't, you could try looking at classifieds in a local paper for a handyperson.

A slant board won't let you do a complete upside-down inversion but it will give you a gentle incline that is actually better for many people.

Instructions

You will need:

- ➤ 6ft x ½" or ⅝" plywood (7ft if you are taller than 6ft).
- ➤ 4 x 3ft of 2x2 timber plus 2 x 6ft of 2x2 (softwood or hardwood, but the fewer knots in the wood, the better).
- ➤ 9ft x 4ft carpet to cover.
- ➤ Screws and carpet tacks.
- ➤ PVA glue.
- ➤ Saw.
- ➤ Screwdriver.
- ➤ Hammer.
- ➤ *Sharp* utility knife.

START THE FRAME

Cut two lengths of the 2x2 softwood to 6ft in length. Cut halving joints at each end (see illustration).

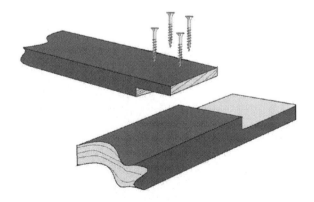

Tee halving joints at the halfway point and 2ft either side of the mid-point. Butt joints can also be used but I would recommend the extra strength of a tee halving joint. I would also recommend using glue as well as screws to secure the joints.

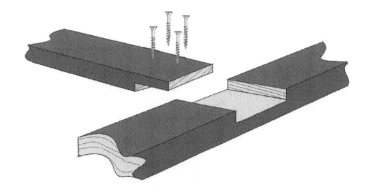

Once this has been done, you will have built what is commonly known as a 'ladder frame' which will support the plywood top.

Now take the sheet of plywood. Fasten it to the framework that you have just built with 1" screws. I would suggest not using glue here as you may need to replace the board should it become worn.

Sand or plane any overhanging plywood to remove any sharp edges which would damage the covering.

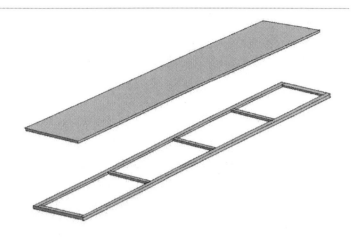

Covering The Board

Take the carpet and place it upside down on the floor or - should you be lucky enough to have one - your workbench.

Place the frame, plywood side down, onto the carpet as shown in the illustration.

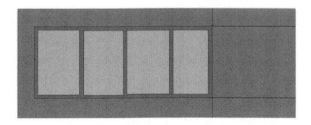

There should be an approximately 18" border all around the board at this stage. Make two cuts as shown and remove both corner pieces.

Repeat at the other end so that you are left with the fabric looking like the illustration below.

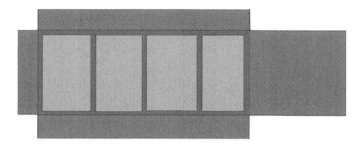

Fold the carpet over on each side of the frame and fasten every 2" with carpet tacks. I suggest carpet tacks as they are less likely to pull through the carpet used but still grip the timber strongly enough to hold the fabric in place. Once all three sides have been done, the underside of the board should look like the illustration below.

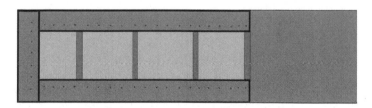

The board is now ready for use!

The flap of material at the top of the board is designed to be tucked under the cushion of an armchair, this holds the board at a good angle and prevents it from sliding out while you use it. If you can get someone to sit on the armchair while you invert, you'll feel even more secure. My large Rough Collie dog comes in useful for this – and it provides entertainment for him as he thinks I look funny upside down.

Should you wish to adapt this design, for example, to fold for storage, it is ***essential*** that any hinge is attached on the underneath of the board. In this way, when the board is folded out and in use, the weight of the person using the board will be pushing the hinge closed, otherwise, the board would simply fold up under the slightest load.

I would also recommend that if this adaptation is considered, 'bar hinges' are employed as they are the only sort I would suggest are capable of handling the weight of even the average adult.

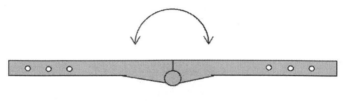

BAR HINGE

And there you have it. A simple home-made slant board that will last years and give you pleasure and health benefits.

FAQ

ෆ✦ఴ

PEOPLE TEND TO HAVE LOTS OF QUESTIONS about inversion therapy. Perhaps because it looks so odd to see someone hanging upside down. Perhaps because they're worried they will develop bat-like characteristics!

Here are some of the questions that I get asked frequently when people discover that it's one of my regular health habits.

How Often Should I Invert?

As long as your physician has no objections to you inverting, you can invert every day – up to twice a day – if you want to. Frequency is an issue when you are first starting with inversion, though. Build up slowly and gradually.

How Long Should I Invert?

Start slowly – give just a minute or two per inversion session. I know it is tempting to try to stay upside down for longer, especially once you've read all the benefits that inversion brings, but please don't. You'll end up with a whopping headache and possibly sinus pain.

Just do a couple of minutes each time for the first few days, to give your brain and body chance to adapt to your new habit.

What's The Best Angle For Inverting?

You start getting the benefits at 20°. 60° is the angle that gives the maximum decompression of the spinal disks. On an inversion table, 60° is the angle where you're lined up with the back legs of the table.

Is It Normal To Feel A Bit Weird Afterwards?

A bit buzzy and energized, yes. A little red in the face, yes.

If you have a headache or sinus pain, or even unusual back ache, you have inverted a bit too long, aim for a shorter time next time. Sit still until the feeling passes and get medical help if it continues.

Does Inversion Increase Blood Pressure?

It can do, temporarily, in the same way that exercise does. That's why you really should avoid it if you have high blood pressure.

It can actually lower your blood pressure eventually because of the relaxation effect, so you don't need to worry about accidentally giving yourself high blood pressure.

APPENDIX 1

WHAT TO DO
IF YOU CAN'T INVERT

ᘓᘏ

IF YOU ARE A FAN OF INVERSION AND BECOME unable to do it – perhaps because of pregnancy or a newly-diagnosed health condition – you will probably miss it a great deal.

Or perhaps you've never been allowed to try inversion – on physician's orders. It is frustrating but if your doctor thinks full inversion could harm you it really isn't worth trying it.

However, there are a few things you can do to alleviate pressure on your spine. As always, check with a health professional first before trying any of these suggestions.

Legs Up The Wall

I was advised to do this by a midwife when I was pregnant, when I was suffering swollen ankles and an aching back. She told me to lie in this position for 10 minutes after work every night. It worked a treat.

It works a bit like inversion therapy by reversing the effects of gravity on the legs. The heart has a tough time pumping blood down to the feet and back up again. Giving it a helping hand by lying with the legs up yet supported brings relief and it even restores energy.

This position can ease back ache, leg ache, swollen ankles, and stress.

Sit/Stand Up

I've mentioned the pressure on the disks of the spine numerous times throughout this book. That pressure is always there, even when lying down, but one of the worst things for increasing it is *leaning forward* while sitting or standing. That makes the usual 10-15lbs that the head weighs feel more like 20-40lbs – depending on how far you lean forward. It puts a tremendous amount of pressure on the muscles and joints of the neck and shoulders. So it's important to sit up when you're sitting down!

> ➢ Try not to slouch forward while sitting at a computer. Sit up or ever so slightly backwards for the least impact on your disks. Move the

monitor and keyboard closer to you so you don't have to lean to see/reach them.

➤ If you have to sit for long periods, get up every hour at a minimum, walk around a bit, do a few stretches. If you can, alter the seat position of your chair every so often.

➤ When standing, keep your head up. It often leans forward, taking the back with it.

➤ You can ease pressure on your back when standing by resting one foot on something – about a brick's height is idea.

➤ If you play sports that require you to lean forwards – e.g. tennis and bowling – try to spend 10 minutes lying down afterwards to decompress the spine.

➤ Never lean forward to pick something or someone up. I'm guilty of this with my little dog, who often wants to be picked up.[43] I'm still at an age where I can bend with my knees but if you aren't, come up with other ways to avoid leaning forward. There are tools[44] to help you pick small items up (the manufacturers say up to 8lbs in weight but in practice it's best to pick up lighter things than that). They are great for picking up things you have dropped, clothes off the floor or out of the washing machine, etc.

There are some great downloadable sheets[45] that show the best positions for sitting while working at a desk

---

[43] I got around it by teaching him to jump!
[44] http://amzn.com/B0000V0AGS
[45] http://www.asd.co.uk/guides/how_to_posters.htm#download

and/or computer. We see health & safety posters all the time but often don't take any notice of them until something goes wrong. By improving our posture, we can not only prevent things going wrong, we can go a long way towards correcting things that already have deteriorated.

Swim

Swimming is a no-impact exercise that enables exercise without any pressure on the joints. Just lying back and floating in the water can be very soothing and relaxing. The water supports the body and reduces the effects of gravity, which means less of a load on the spine.

Some experts caution against using the breaststroke if you have back problems. That's because many people swim with their head up, causing an unnatural tilt backwards of the neck. Keep that up for a half-hour swim and you could end up with neck pain, dizziness, and worse.

If you love breaststroke, the way around the neck strain problem is simply to wear swimming goggles. They will enable you to lie flat in the water (face-down), rather than straining your neck backwards. You will have to come up for air, obviously, but if you put your feet down while you do so, you will keep your body unit more 'together' and reduce the strain on your neck.

Don't Hold Your Breath

The European Spine Journal[46] highlighted the fact that people with chronic lower back pain tend to have altered breathing patterns.

Dr Stuart McGill from the University of Waterloo has proved that there is extra pressure in the abdomen when holding the breath and that can help to stabilize the lumbar region of the back. So that seems like a good idea but it isn't because it increases the pressure in the disks of the spine.

The body's instinct to protect the lower back is correct but if we habitually hold our breath we are putting unnecessary extra pressure on our spinal disks.

The lesson here is to be aware of your breathing when performing any activity.

I try not to repeat myself in my books but this is so important and ground-breathing that I'm going to add some [cut-down] information here about Linda Stone's work from my skin brushing book. Apologies if you've read that one!

Linda Stone is a highly respected writer and trend consultant who became aware that she routinely held her breath while checking her email. She watched to see if others did the same and they do[47]. She noticed it

---

[46] http://link.springer.com/article/10.1007%2Fs00586-009-1020-y#page-2

[47] http://www.dailymail.co.uk/sciencetech/article-2509391/do-email-apnoea-80-people-stop-breathing-properly-typing.html

mainly among office workers, who frequently held their breath while working. She calls it 'email apnea'.

She asked leading doctors if breath holding and shallow breathing can affect a person's health - especially when done day in, day out. Apparently it really can.

One of the many doctors she consulted with was Dr Margaret Chesney, from the National Institute of Health (NIH). Dr Chesney had proved in her own research with another NIH scientist, Dr David Anderson, that breath holding and hyperventilating (fast breathing) alter the body's oxygen, carbon dioxide, and nitrous oxide balance and contributes *significantly* to stress-related diseases.

HOW TO BREATHE

If you watch a baby breathe you'll see that the movement doesn't involve his little chest, it's his round tummy that goes up and down.

This 23 second video shows it perfectly:

http://bit.ly/babybreathing

Learning to breathe properly will help relax your mind and body and get good oxygen supplies to your whole system. Then it's just a matter of remembering to do it and not hold your breath!

Over the page is a simple routine to learn how to breathe properly.

Simple Breathing Routine

Lie on your back on the floor with your calves resting on something like a coffee table. Your thighs should be vertical, with your knees pointing at the ceiling. Your calves should be horizontal on the coffee table, with your feet relaxed. In this position your shoulders sit in their proper place and your neck, back and abdominal muscles can relax. This will prevent you from using the neck and shoulders when you are breathing, and enable you to learn where you should be breathing from. Stay in this position for a minute or so, just relaxing and becoming aware of your breathing. Try to notice what it is doing without influencing it - not easy!

Put your left hand on your abdomen just over and above your belly button. Take a few slightly longer and deeper breaths than you are used to. Inhale through your nose and exhale through your mouth. The chances are that your hand won't move very much and you may be aware that your chest does. That's fine, for now. As the diaphragm is largely muscle, it gets stronger and more capable the more you exercise it - and it gets weak and floppy when you don't - so we're going to exercise it. Eventually, diaphragmatic breathing will become second-nature to you.

cont/d ...

Inhale and think about your diaphragm (which is beneath your hand) expanding downwards. Focus on drawing your breath in low into the base of your lungs, where your diaphragm is making room for their expansion by easing your ribs out to the sides. Do this over a slow count of 4. Hold it for just a couple of seconds but don't close your throat, stay relaxed, and then...

Exhale (slowly, through your mouth) and think about your diaphragm beginning to rise again as your lungs release air and your ribs relax back into place. Exhale over a slow count of 4. You can slightly draw in your abdomen if it helps.

Importantly, don't take another deep breath, just relax and allow your breathing to go back to normal. Most deep breathing exercises don't do this, they get you to do lots of deep breaths together, which can be a bit overwhelming for a body that isn't used to all that oxygen.

After half a minute or so, take another deep breath.

The more you do this, the more likely it is that it will become natural and something you will eventually do without thinking about.

∽∾

So, as you have seen, there are quite a few things you can do to really benefit your health and make up for the fact that you can't do inversion. Just remembering to breathe could have huge benefits.

APPENDIX 2

CELEBRITIES WHO USE INVERSION THERAPY

ᏟᏒᎦᎦᏩᎧ

THERE ARE A NUMBER OF CELEBRITIES WHO have realized the value of inversion. I'm not particularly a celebrity watcher but I find it very encouraging that these people who are at the height of their earning ability choose something as simple as inversion to keep themselves healthy.

A blockbuster actor loses millions of dollars if he can't appear in a movie because of a bad back so it is important that he uses preventative methods to keep healthy. There are other reasons that celebrities use inversion therapy as well.

Dan Brown

The bestselling author of *The Da Vinci Code* hangs upside down to help him write. He told a British newspaper[48] about his technique of seeking inspiration when he struggles with writer's block.

> *"It does help. You've just got to relax and let go. The more you do it the more you let go. And then soon it's just, wow."*
>
> Dan Brown, author

He uses various methods for inverting, including an inversion table and gravity boots.

Eva Mendes

The actress looked amazing in the hit film *Hitch* (with Will Smith). Some of it may be due to her practice of inversion therapy.

She says[49] she lies upside down on a slant board for 20 minutes before photo shoots. She does it to increase blood flow to her upper body and face, to give her a vibrant look.

---

[48] http://bit.ly/danbrowninversion
[49] http://www.wellsphere.com/skin-health-article/eva-mendes-headstand-for-anti-aging/460908

Sheri-Ann Brooks

Olympic athlete Sheri-Ann Brooks is reported on the Teeter Fitness website[50] as saying that inversion helps both her performance and recovery after events. She believes:

> **"Inversion therapy helps reduce muscle tension and the likelihood of ligament strains."**
>
> Sheri-Ann Brooks, Olympic athlete

Rosie O'Donnell

Comedian Rosie O'Donnell claimed on an episode of *The View* that she uses inversion therapy as a way to control her depression. There don't appear to have been any studies done into inversion therapy's ability to help depression but that just means no-one saw a way of making enough money out of it to make funding a study worthwhile.

I would guess that the relaxation and circulation boosting effects of inversion could have some influence on mood.

There could also be some connection with the 'second brain' in the gut. More serotonin (the hormone that

---

[50] http://www.teeter-fitness.com/

Prozac works on) is made in the gut than in the brain. We know that inversion relieves pressure on the internal organs, especially the transverse (cross-body) colon, which can sag. I wonder if that is the reason that Ms O'Donnell is experiencing some relief? Possibly.

Numerous other celebrities are reportedly enjoying the benefits of inversion therapy but I was unable to find original sources. Inversion manufacturers report that the following celebrities are fans of inversion:

- ➢ Jackie Chan
- ➢ David Duchovny
- ➢ Martha Stewart
- ➢ Gene Simmons
- ➢ David Blaine
- ➢ Uri Geller
- ➢ Steve Truglia (Daniel Craig's James Bond stuntman)
- ➢ Rock band 311

SOURCES &
FURTHER READING

ര‍ജ‍ഇ‍ാ

Books

Broad, William J., *The Science of Yoga: The Risks and the Rewards*. Simon & Schuster. 2012

Gonzalez, Carlos M, *Hanging Out for the Health of It: One Minute a Day to a Happier, Healthier, & Longer Life*. Advantage Media Group. 2008

Jonsson, Egon & Nachemson, A.L., *Neck & Back Pain: The Scientific Evidence of Causes, Diagnosis, & Treatment*. Lippincott Williams & Wilkins. 2000.

Kapandji, I A, MD, *The Physiology of the Joints, Volume III*. Churhill Livingstone. 2008.

Martin, Robert M, *The Gravity Guiding System*. Gravity Guidance, Inc. 1982.

Nachemson, Alf, et al: *Intravital Dynamic Pressure Measurements in Lumbar Discs*. 1970

Russell, Peter, The Brain Book. Routledge & Kegan Paul. 1979.

Thomas, Hugh O, *Diseases of the Hip, Knee, & Ankle Joints*. Jeremy Norman Co. Collectors edition 1991.

Research Studies

Alf Nachemson's numerous studies on spinal health:

*http://www.ncbi.nlm.nih.gov/pubmed/?term=
Nachemson%20AL[Author]&cauthor=
true&cauthor_uid=7209680*

Inversion Therapy: A Study of Physiological Effects. Vernon, Howard, BA, DC, FCCS(C), Meschino, James, DC, Naiman, Joseph, DC. Available from the National Institutes of Health:

*http://www.ncbi.nlm.nih.gov/pmc/articles/
PMC2484360/pdf/jcca00075-0029.pdf*

Inversion therapy in patients with pure single level lumbar discogenic disease: a pilot randomized trial. Prasad, KS, Gregson, BA, Hargreaves, G, Byrnes, T, Winburn P, Mendelow, AD.

*http://www.ncbi.nlm.nih.gov/pubmed/
22263648*

Magazines & Journal Articles

'The Effects of Inversion Traction on Spinal Column Configuration, Heart Rate, Blood Pressure, & Perceived Discomfort', Ballantyne, Byron T, BA, PT, Reser, Michael D, BS, PT, Lorenza, G William, BS, PT, Smidt, Gary L, PhD, PT. The Journal of Orthopedic & Sports Physical Therapy. 1986.

http://www.jospt.org/doi/pdf/10.2519/
jospt.1986.7.5.254

'Altered breathing patterns during lumbopelvic motor control tests in chronic low back pain: a case-control study', Roussel, Nathalie, Nijs, Jo, Truijen, Steven, Vervecken, Liesbet, Mottram, Sarah, Stassijns, Gaetane. European Spine Journal. 2009.

http://link.springer.com/article/
10.1007%2Fs00586-009-1020-y#page-2

Other References

WHAT IS INVERSION THERAPY?

http://www.spine-health.com/conditions/spine-anatomy/back-muscles-and-low-back-pain

BENEFITS OF INVERSION THERAPY

Pros and cons of inversion tables:

*http://www.livestrong.com/article/
31503-pros-cons-inversion-tables/*

How a Teeter inversion table decompresses your spine:

*http://www.youtube.com/
watch?v=7c2f5NaEuZM*

12 health benefits of inversions:

*http://www.bewellbuzz.com/wellness-
buzz/inversions/*

New discoveries of additional inversion therapy benefits found:

*http://www.prweb.com/releases/2012/3/
prweb9345588.htm*

NEGATIVE EFFECTS OF INVERSION THERAPY

Negative effects of inversion therapy on Livestrong:

*http://www.livestrong.com/article/112991-
negative-effects-inversion-therapy/*

OTHER HEALTH NOTES

Height loss with age:

*http://www.nlm.nih.gov/medlineplus/
ency/article/003998.htm*

THE 10-DAY SKIN BRUSHING DETOX CHAPTER EXCERPT

ⱽⱽ

D id you like *Inversion Therapy*? If you are interested in health and wellness, you may like dry skin brushing. It's an incredible, easy, inexpensive naturopathic technique that you can incorporate into your daily routine.

Here's a free excerpt from *The 10-Day Skin Brushing Detox* book.

HOW SKIN BRUSHING CAN REVOLUTIONIZE YOUR HEALTH

DESPITE BEING A fan of dry skin brushing, I laughed at the spa episode of the *Rosanne* TV show with everyone else in 1996. The episode was called 'Pampered to a Pulp' and portrayed skin brushing as an activity more suited to a torture chamber than a health spa.

I had qualified as an aromatherapist and massage therapist the year before, gaining diplomas from the International Institute of Health & Holistic Therapies and doing further study in nutrition (the nutrition courses were just out of interest, not to professional level).

None of my courses had covered skin brushing but my training made me realize that it would have many of the benefits of massage, plus some more, be quick and easy to do, and - unlike massage - would be easy to do yourself, without someone else doing the work.

I did experience the excellent results that skin brushing brings, but also suffered unfortunate side-effects. I couldn't find out any information about them, either online or in books or scientific papers. So I gave up daily brushing and just brushed occasionally.

When clients asked about skin brushing, I always advised them to be very careful. Brushing a healthy body is fine but when people with pre-existing illnesses take up brushing, they often become overwhelmed with negative side-effects.

A few years ago, I researched Manual Lymphatic Drainage (MLD). A close friend was battling cancer and MLD can help some of the painful swelling that can happen after lymph gland removal. I wanted to find out more about it before helping her find a therapist.

Now, if you read anything about skin brushing, the instructions will almost always say to start at the feet and work up, always brushing towards the heart. Some advise quite vigorous brushing. But MLD therapists don't start at the feet and they always use very gentle movements. Discovering that made a light bulb go off over my head! I had been doing skin brushing wrong for years.

Over a couple of months, I devised my own method, based on MLD principles and the effects I noticed. Then I started getting the people I massaged to try my method. They loved it and found that the effects spurred them on to continue brushing and to implement lifestyle changes.

There is no need for anyone to suffer with skin brushing and I'll show you how to take up the habit without succumbing to overwhelming side-effects that make you want to give up. You will find that skin brushing can kick-start a healthier lifestyle, because it gives you a glow, energy, and a new vibrancy that carries through into the rest of your life.

If you choose to *add* healthy foods, drinks, and habits to your life, instead of focusing on removing things, you will have an attitude of enjoyment and lack of stress. That feeling makes you feel WELL. Giving up stuff doesn't make you feel good; it puts your body into an alert mode, warning it that there's possible stress coming. The body starts putting stores of food into fat cells for later use, in case of famine; it cuts down on non-essential processes (such as copious energy, glossy hair, strong nails) and focuses on basic survival.

Natural energy – energy that comes from eating food that gives you nutrients, not food that uses them up – is amazing. It is nothing like the fake energy you get from chocolate or coffee. For a start, it lasts longer and doesn't leave you feeling even worse when the effects wear off because they don't wear off. There's also a kind of serenity that comes with natural energy that is hard to describe.

This skin brushing detox plan works as a type of diet because:

> ➤ Your new glow will make you feel less like cramming a whole chocolate cake into your mouth or reaching for your third glass of wine.

> ➤ You won't want to lose the healthy buzz so your body won't crave the old junk foods that used to give you a temporary lift but then a depressing fall-off.

> ➤ If you follow my recommendations about diet you will possibly be eating more than usual and that will make you feel less deprived, less stressed, and more at peace. You are far less likely to crave calorie dense, stodgy foods that feel like a lead lump in your stomach and sap your energy.

> ➤ You will be more relaxed and less stressed because you're doing something beneficial for your body.

> ➤ Dieting *isn't* the way to lose weight. Detoxing isn't either. The only way to lose weight is to get healthy. A healthy body has no need of emergency stores of food, conveniently packaged in fat cells.

This book is about abundance and enjoyment. It's about taking up a new, enjoyable habit that makes you feel wonderful and then easing in some new health choices to support and nourish your mind and body.

It's about turning the word 'detox' on its head, realizing that we don't need to deprive ourselves in order to help our bodies go about their natural detoxification routines.

10 days are enough to give your body's natural detoxification systems a helping hand and to start you on the skin brushing habit. I was going to use the word 'addiction' instead of habit there, because that's what it's like. You feel so great that you won't want to miss a day!

After the 10 days, you could introduce another new habit or perhaps give up an old unhelpful habit, again for another 10 days. The 10 days thing is important because it takes that time for your body to adapt, to start to make it a habit, and to avoid clashing cleansing reactions. If you gave up caffeine, you'd probably get headaches. But if you gave up caffeine at the same time as taking up weight training, you couldn't be sure if it was the lack of caffeine or perhaps a pulled muscle in your neck causing the headaches.

You may not need a vast improvement in your health, you may just want a bit of a boost or smoother skin. Great. Long may it continue. It still applies that it is less stressful for your body if you take up new things one at a time though. If you have done skin brushing before you can just use this book to learn my new method and hopefully pick up some other tips as well.

The main thing I hope you will get out of this book is this:

GO EASY

I'm pretty sure you won't believe me though, as skin brushing seems so simple and inoffensive. That's why the *Introduction* of this book goes into more detail about what happens when we deprive our bodies and *Chapter 1: My Story* details the side-effects that I experienced when I took up skin brushing. If you don't like personal stories then please feel free to skip it and go to *Chapter 2: A New Technique*.

Let's get started with a closer look at detoxing…

The 10-Day Skin Brushing Detox is available from Amazon and good bookstores. You may even be able to order it from your local library!

INDEX

☙❧

ABOUT THE AUTHOR

MIA CAMPBELL, I.I.H.H.T., IS AN EXPERIENCED aromatherapist and health coach. She was born in Lancashire in the UK and until recently treated private clients in the North-West of England.

She was badly injured in a car accident and determined to learn natural therapies to help rebuild her own health and teach others.

Mia enjoys playing and writing music, field archery, and swimming. She is passionate about animal welfare and has a house full of rescued animals – some of whom found their own way there!

She recently returned from an extended road trip in an RV around the US, Canada, & Mexico and is currently writing a book based on the trip.

Made in the USA
San Bernardino, CA
02 December 2018